Depression
Let's Kick
its Ass

I0093224

By
Jen MacVicar

Copyright © 2025 Jen Macvicar
All Rights Reserved

Table of Contents

Chapter 1:
Depression let's kick its ass

I woke up today and decided today was the day I shared my darkest secrets, my most inner fears and why, and most importantly, how Depression has controlled my life since I was a little girl. I am now a 54-year-old daughter, mother, and grandma who has lived with Depression and PTSD for over 30 years.

Over my life I have had challenges both small and life-changing. Growing up, or becoming older as each year passed, was harder to deal with. In some instances, still wanting to live was the hardest challenge I kept facing and will continue to face as I go through life just as you reading this will. As hard as I have fallen and as hard as it was to get back up, I will continue to strive to put one foot in front of the other and continue to stand back up for the sake of my children and my beautiful grand babies.

Only my closest friends know that I suffer from depression. If you were to walk in my office or into my house and meet me, you would never know. I believe if you asked a person who suffers from Depression which they would rather have:

1. Depression
2. Disability
3. Anything of your choosing.

Depression is the hardest, most unbearable disease one can have. There is no cure; there is no real solution to correct the imbalance in one's brain function. If there was sign me up for sure. I know for the last 30 years of my life I have done a magnificent job hiding my emotions. But also, at times I have lost it and have had suicidal thoughts that I have an extremely challenging time getting out of my head. After so long of dealing with and trying to hide and submerge these emotions, sometimes they win. The amount you win and lose becomes the game of life when you have depression.

As hard as my journey has been, I have fought to win, even with this last devastation I am presently having to deal with. When someone doesn't have the dreadful imbalance, they do not understand that some joys become crushing factors and could leave one on a very thin line of survival.

In each chapter I will walk you through the journey of depression through my heartache and downfalls. Please realize that after each chapter I get back up from my falls and try life again. Life I have learned is not about how easy life is, but how you handle it and bring forth the best you can under any circumstance. By the end, I am not looking for anyone to feel bad for me and my life. I am hoping, with my story, that I can help another understand that they are not the only ones; that they too can find inner peace at some point in their lives.

Inner peace doesn't always mean you will have peace from the effects of depression, but you can become the success of your own story in life. Depression will never go away as we are told, there will never ever be a cure! The cure for one's imbalance of thoughts, fears, and simple things in life has not been found. You need to believe that you can one day control all your fears. You just need to realize that you are strong enough to take control. Remember there will always be new and frightful fears that enter all our lives. It's how we control our emotions and fight back with our physical being. Believe me, over time it does get better. It is only you who can make the choice to change. We as individuals have the freedom to make those options come to life. Through extremely challenging work and by taking baby steps to change, things will change.

Depression

What does depression really mean for most of us? For every person it means a different set of circumstances that have brought on a whole new set of uncontrollable emotions and a lifetime of confusion. For some it is stemmed from the smallest incident in their lives; for others, from a very pronounced chain reaction in life. For some it's been a lifetime struggle from a young age, and for a great deal of us who suffer, it makes life so much more challenging.

Most experts, for a long time, passed off childhood depression when I was growing up, and the doctor I saw always chalked it up to me just wanting attention. Yeah, in some ways that is what she must have felt… I was also the middle child of five: two adoptions and two biological siblings, not to mention our parents bringing in foster children from time to time. For me, I truly had depression. I was not 13 seeing this doctor. By this time for years I was being physically molested by two cousins and a babysitter. Then, because the doctor said I was faking it, my parents never listened. They never gave me so much as ten minutes to talk.

The only time they paid any attention was if I acted out in a bad way. Then at least I got noticed. Other than that, I always knew in my heart I was the black sheep of the family. Not just with my immediate family all the uncles and aunties always felt the same way, except for only one aunty and one uncle; those two I have always treasured and always will.

If you are to sit with someone with depression, would you know if the person next to you suffered from depression? I can say no it's almost impossible to see on the surface of a person. For most who suffer from depression it is both an emotional and physical challenge every day. Any person I have come across will chalk my mood up to being tired, having a difficult day, or constantly being told to get over it! Depression is not something anybody discusses for a great many reasons:

- People with depression really understand the magnitude of feeling lost.

- People don't understand that it is a chemical imbalance in the brain and in one's soul.

- Having depression, for me, is an embarrassment: that they are not in control of their emotions, their self-worth, their self-esteem. The whole body becomes suppressed with pain.

- People with depression have become the best actors/actresses out there. They are the first to hide the disease and the first to act as if they are in the best of spirits and moods despite a constant battle of emotions.

- People with depression suffer in every part of who they are the emotional roller coaster that never seems to stop.

- The pain caused by depression increases with each depressive episode or with increases in emotional or physical incidents.

- The hardest part is the mental anguish depression gives to people: the thought of being a failure, never being what your family expected you to be or do. The deepest emotional fight we never leave is the one that becomes our forever battle in life. It is very sad when this one wins against the good fight you are trying to conquer. I was a teenager when I tried twice and failed both times to let it win. Just recently my much younger cousin suffered she tried, and now I never get to see her. My heart broke when I heard the sad news.

There isn't a day that goes by that I don't hear it from someone: "You are so happy are you always such a morning person?" If they only knew the actual struggles I face every day just trying to get out of bed and get on with my day. When you suffer from depression it hits you in so many different ways it becomes unbearable for some. Unfortunately, that is when the evil of the disease wins. Those are the days when the struggle is even harder; for some it's the day that happens to end it all.

Have I personally thought of taking my life? I believe more people than we know have. Depression is exhausting; it is physically draining to both the body and the mind. Even decades later after my first try, I would still say I have had those thoughts, but I have never acted on them since. It took a great deal of hard work to not be so selfish. It is a quick solution but not the correct one. The destruction that is caused by suicide only leaves a lifetime of unanswered questions for the ones left behind.

Back in the early years when I was growing up they spoke about this as much as they did for people who were absolutely completely comfortable being gay. Both were so harshly looked at. It forced some of us with depression even deeper into our rabbit hole. Talking or having someone to talk to back then well, there just wasn't any place or anyone to help us. Not only did I suffer really young on way too many incidents, I had to always keep my mouth shut.

I am happy to see and hear there are now places or people that are available to talk. Even the hotlines we didn't have back then. Remember: no one can help unless you ask for help. No one knows about your heartbreak and depression. Keeping it inside left me with medical issues for my entire life.

Asking yeah right! That is what I thought too. I still don't have someone who would be me who would understand why I was such a bad kid. I was fucken bad for good reason and not a soul seen, not a soul led me a hand. I never knew what a shoulder to cry on meant. I still don't. But I have learned I have less heartache being long. I am long into my life. I chose to be alone to enjoy my life for what is left. I want to live on my terms. I don't need any more judgement. I still get that from my family.

Taking control isn't going to be easy. And if someone says it is, they absolutely have no fuckin idea the damage they can do mentally, physically, emotionally and spiritually. As I sit here and think about what I am writing I have a sense that I need to address actual issues that hinder us daily with depression. Yes, taking things too far because you just can't do it anymore... pause, breathe. Remember: I believe in you.

Writing, I am reminded of the ones I have lost the ones I have lots of friends. Family. The heartache looking at news on TV saying so and so... You sit there stunned because you never had guessed they suffered. You are not the only one on this journey; there are others just waiting for your reaching hand.

I remember suffering in the darkness of each day being silent. When I was young well, before we made the big move to a town I fell off a cliff on a summer day. There were a bunch of us that used to hike in our town. As we were hiking we came across a view like you have never seen. We looked down and we could see a perfect place we could have our picnic at.

Of course, I was the smallest so they lifted me down. They say "ready, set," they let go!!! I didn't stop. I fell 45 feet down to the bottom. I didn't remember the fall, I didn't remember getting home either. My head hurt so bad, so did my body. I wasn't able to remember, so my parents never knew about the fall. From that day I didn't remember any of my deepest fears. I literally had no memory of even that last week. I had a feeling of loss but I didn't know what it was. I tried to talk to my parents but they were always too busy with everyone else.

Shortly after we moved to another town got uprooted with really no explanation. A month or so passed and my mother says the babysitter is going to watch the younger ones after school and get them off to school. OK, went to school and when I walked through the door a feeling of uncertainty, a deep emotional feeling was taking control of my entire body.

I walked into the living room and our babysitter from our last town was now living a few blocks away. Deep inside me I felt a feeling of wanting to run away. Within days this man had me pinned in my bedroom. He sexually abused me right there. He put his hands down my pants and rubbed his body against me. I pushed away. I said no, but… it went unheard. It went down so deep inside me I couldn't cry. I froze. I lost myself that day.

It was decades later when my memories came flushing back I then realized I was twice robbed of my innocence. I was robbed of and thrown to the side. No one ever listened to my cries. No one even noticed how destroyed emotionally and mentally I was only 13. Twice this man took everything from me with no hesitation on his part.

He used his knowledge and his power over me to convince me this was the right thing we were doing. He convinced me he loved me, that he wanted just me, that he would love me forever. The only thing I wanted as a child was to be loved someone offering to love me. Not knowing any better I gave in. So, whenever he wanted to, he did, right where we was.

For the next eight months any chance he had to babysit or offer to tutor me, he did. Back then there was no one to talk to, no one to trust. By this point in my life I started hating myself; I hated living. I had such an emotional breakdown and had no one to turn to. It left me hindered as my life still moved forward. Finally, one day it stopped without any warning. My mom says he went across Canada.

I was once again left alone. The fear was building up as my mother continued to talk. Her words fell silent. I couldn't hear her; my world was closing in. I had never had this powerful pain in my chest I couldn't get a breath of air. I felt betrayed. I felt that now I am so damaged no one would love me.

The damage was already done; my earlier years still were not part of my being then. As I learned way later, that he was already raping me much younger than I was. It was like living it all over again. I became angry. I stayed that way for years to come. My anger became my friend. It kept people away from me so I didn't have to lose anyone again. More so… I kept my wall up because no one was ever going to do that to me again.

Damn it was New Year's Eve and I was late for curfew, not by much, but my father decided to ground me, punished me right in front of all their guests. Then my older sister came home. She comes in my room and says, "I am pregnant what am I supposed to do?" Man, I was shocked; I was completely stunned. As she was sitting beside me our father walked into the bedroom and gave me shit for my sister being in there!

WTF, right? I was pissed. My father was accusing me of being a slut because I was late getting home. More to the fact like, fuck I was sleeping around. My father always accused me of that. My blood boiled as I was being raped almost daily and you say I am a slut? I yelled, "Well I am not pregnant my sister was!" No shit my father stopped in his shoes then grounded me even longer. Even today that incident pisses me the fuck off. I never got an apology ever no matter how many times my father was wrong.

I found growing up that the little things are what set off my depression. For years I spiraled out of control. Most of my teenage years were a blur. My depression hindered my emotional development and my ability to stop my thoughts of loneliness and emptiness. Living with depression when I was growing up, I do understand why more people did think they just wanted to end their suffering. I know firsthand how hard that fight to stay alive is. I still fight it, but I fight now with better knowledge I have a better understanding. And no, I still do not have family around. Well I do, but I am the black sheep so absolutely no invites.

Life just seemed as if everything was going wrong. My parents were splitting up due to my mom's final chance. I can't remember how many chances our father gave her to change, to get off those pills. My dad probably put her in rehab five or six times. It never worked. She stayed addicted until her passing. Oh my my parents used to fight. Back then husbands had different rights according to the law… back then husbands had a right, yes, to hit the wives and more importantly, which was the ultimate punishment: he was allowed to rape his wife. It was classified as wifely duties. Yup later on you will read me addressing this very same issue in my own life circumstance.

At times I stop and think really hard if I want to talk about the next event or incident, as some dumb ass stated to me once. I never say, "You want to walk in my shoes?" I don't because I wouldn't want this turmoil in anyone's life. The heartbreak, the emotional breakdown of yourself. I have walked a thousand miles more than I ever needed to.

Time for a laugh… it is needed. So, my mom would always get stoned on her pills then go shopping for groceries. Now there were eight kids and two adults so weekly shopping was required. But my mother always writes a cheque before my dad's pay. So, one day she went shopping and got like $900. The manager at the store called the bank they said no money. He got in his truck, went right to our place.

I was just getting home and he just stopped yelling at my mom! "I am here to take these backs. I am sick and fucken tired of bounced cheques." My chin literally hit the ground. Is Todd there stunned and watched him load all the groceries in his truck. Well damn my father got home as he was getting out his truck. He got out, came and told my father and I never seen someone laugh so hard; he

12

shook the man's hand. I still laugh at that even today. The day before I had the last laugh I would have in a real long time.

Went to school and instead of going to our classes we were sent to our homerooms. The school was silent; there were no kids talking. It seemed that quite a few of our friends were not here. We sat down and the teachers walked in. As she gathered her composure tears filled her eyes. The words came out that we lost five school children last night in a fire. They are all students from high school.

You can hear the cries of some students and you can hear the loudness of the crying. We were all told that there would be counseling here if you need it. We were sent home. The next day coming to class was hard. All five of them hung out at the same doors as me. I had already dealt with some death before this but this one hit home being jive growing teenagers. So many students kept leaving throughout the day. The overwhelming sense of sadness and loss.

My heart hurt my soul, the devastation of the ones left behind, the friends in deep despair. Watching so much devastation was hard to see for some so hard to understand. Questions I am sure are even asked today: How did they not get out? The windows were boarded up and something fell in front of the door. The smoke filled the house; they had no way out. They were holding each other's hands.

As the days passed we listened to the stories being told. We listened to the anger of "why?" That kind of trauma never leaves; it is always there. Their decision to make a fire to stay warm was the very thing that took all their lives. Five young lives lost that day. The trauma lasts a lifetime for some. Trauma that is intense will always be in your mind. It is up to you to channel that fear.

I had to go to the funeral of a fellow classmate who lost his battle with depression. I saw the anguished faces of his family and friends.

It was an open casket and it scared the living hell out of me. I have never forgotten my friend's face that day. Seeing the pain in his mother's heart, as I watched her go from person to person, she was unbelievable. She wanted all of us friends to be okay. She wasn't mad at his passing; she understood, even though he kept his depression a deep, dark secret. I thought to myself, *man, I want her power to handle bad situations.*

What I observed, going through the loss of friends and watching a broken mother deal with the heartbreak that was before her, was this: healing, I believe, is the moment you decide to take the first step towards it. It is not always easy and it certainly doesn't happen overnight, but with each new day you are moving closer to the peace you deserve.

Healing is about understanding that it is okay to feel broken sometimes, but it's also knowing that you are strong enough to rebuild. It's about forgiving yourself, letting go of the past, and embracing the future. You will climb up, but you will also fall down. Pull yourself up and try it is all you can do. Believe in yourself and have faith.

Through all my battles I have had in life, I am still here. I still take a breath every day, even when it seems like I can't. I work harder for every breath and every step I take that day. Yeah, it might take your pain away, but what is left is the pain and suffering of the ones who lost you. The turmoil suicide causes is that you jeopardize your loved ones' well-being. You leave them with no answers on why you chose not to fight. You add more pain and suffering. You leave questions that forever go through everyone's minds. It becomes the very thing that can drive people into depression. It is your choice that determines your family's ability to handle your departure. It really isn't the answer to any problem, because that problem you had now becomes the families.

Your actions solve absolutely nothing. You take away your mother's loving touch and your family's ability to spend your life with you. You rob your children of a father or a mother. Depression is like a boxing match: you will always have a next round, but it is only up to you to win each and every one of them. We all need help. It is how we ask and how we take control that determines who wins. Sometimes a bad day is just a bad day. On those other days, get up and say, *fuck you I take control of my day, of my life, of my wanting to live.*

Yes, I can say I have several times over my life tried to commit suicide. What is sad is I am still young. To be so lost, so confused, to have the ultimate loneliness within. As I have watched the best of the best be brought down with depression, some days it's even harder to think, *how the hell am I going to make it if they can't?* What is it that stops me from following through with it? I would say it is when I see the heartache of the people they have left behind. My saving grace was and always will be my grandson he loves his nana, and that is what I need: unconditional love, no matter how I feel.

Over the last few decades I have educated myself on a constant basis to deal with my depression. I have had some good heartfelt laughs reading what people think is the issue. I have read countless papers written about the subject. I have personally been in therapy for years. And yes, I combat my depression with an antidepressant. I have been on them for about 10 years. I will be on them for the rest of my life. Taking medication is not a cure and it is not the solution, but for some it holds back their darkest days and allows them to fight a little easier.

The hardest decision I ever had to make was accepting I had depression and even worse, that I was suffering from added pressure and distress because of PTSD. I always just told myself things were alright. It was just a bad day. But then suddenly I was hit with a wave of uncontrollable emotions that took over. I had

15

countless days of crying, not eating, feeling so overwhelmed I just didn't get out of bed. When you have depression, it takes over your body and mind in so many horrific ways. Some days it's hard just to get the mind to not focus on the pain, the worry, the stress of it all.

When we first have children, we want to shelter them and keep them from harm. No matter how hard some of the best tried, they were unable to shelter some from depression. I am sure when my parents had me their last thought would be that having an unhappy child was the last thing on their mind. It was very prominent in me that I suffered from something young. But what doctors chalked it up to was middle child syndrome! No, it wasn't, but it was far easier than dealing with the truth. It was far easier than accepting that your child was sick. Bad news for most who suffer from depression we get swept under the rug and told to suck it up and be happy. If parents look back now, I am almost sure they would think differently or hopefully at least speak differently to the child.

Unless you personally suffer all the dark areas of depression, you can really never know how that person really feels. Sure, there are enough theories to give advice! There is enough documentation brought to our attention on the struggles of depression. But when a person writes any paper, whether theory or not, it's based on a personal opinion they want us to focus on. How do they focus on helping that individual without implementing a course of action with them? Their course of action is based only on the direction you want it to go. Some papers need to also state other contributing factors to both depression and PTSD.

I was brought up in the '70s and '80s. There was not much discussion on depression as there is now. If you are wondering, no there is not much more new evidence, and evidence is often given solely based around personal objectives rather than the truth behind what it means to have depression. In my day there was no personal chance of surviving depression; it was hidden; it was something

16

they did not touch on if you were a child. Because of me having childhood depression it escalated with age and with each traumatic episode since. I never got the chance to see if it would have ended up different had they seen I was already suffering at a young age.

The hardest struggle we all have that suffer from depression is getting back up again. I know that feeling all too well. I have had more struggles and traumatic events over my years; I swear I can fill two lives easily. But they have all been mine to bear. My journey from where I started to where I am headed has been a very long battle of falling and standing, holding my head up each time. None of my hardship or frustration in life was because of being or having the middle kid syndrome. As I have gone from a fragile innocent little girl to a fragile middle-age woman, I can say it's been a hardship getting to where I am in life. As well, it is still a continued journey that will never end with depression. It will forever be with you. It is how we learn to control it that makes life more meaningful and rewarding.

I believe I have come to the lowest, deepest, darkest days of my life. Well, it's been running for two weeks and there is no light at the end of the tunnel. I know at times I have struggled and had to struggle hard, but this time holy shit I seriously fucked up my own life in so many ways. It has left me homeless, helpless, and more scared than I have even been. All those other issues in my life have not compared to this. Maybe I should believe those downfalls and hiccups in my life were setting me up for my final battle.

I had to lose everything most dear to me; I lost the most important people in my life. I lost my happiness and it has been gone for a very long time. It wasn't until I was sitting outside living on the streets for the night oh how low I had gone how much I have messed up my own life and that of my family once again. I would say I was being put up against a wall for years. My sense of duty to family and friends seemed lost, so out of reach I may never get some of them back. Hold tight to those ones you love the most. Those are the ones who might help you heal.

For just over three years my mind has not been grounded. It seems my rift from wrong was not in the direction it should be. My emotional state had never reached it. Such an overload to my life. I turned into a mean person. I turned my direction to the wrong people. I have hurt people over these last few years. I am so deeply sorry from the bottom of my heart. I should have directed my emotions and actions to the people who put me into believing depression was in my head and that I was only looking for attention. It placed a lifetime of shame on me that I never should have had to endure, constant nightmares, not to mention the lack of self-respect and self-dignity or worth. I got robbed of being a child, being a teenager; I robbed my children of having a better-rounded mother.

God knows I have made tons of mistakes with them. The hardest thing to live with is knowing you are truly alone in this battle. After fighting for years then decades you tend to stop reaching out and you stop growing into the person you should be. The ashamed walls are put up and the isolation of letting people know you suffer now is your own battle. That is when depression wins. Our truths will always hide behind our words; each time we are breaking every day in our own silence. No one ever sees the pain. Even now as I write, I was never "never okay"I learned how to pretend very young. As I am sure you have. My feelings have definitely made me a different person. I am not at all the person I used to be.

My journey has not been easy, and having the lack of support in my early years I didn't have the options to talk about it. In time I became quieter, more careful with each new upset; I became harder to reach. I know I have and always have love in my heart now, just not for the ones who have used and abused me. It is up to ourselves to protect our peace. I wish I knew that growing up. Remove yourself immediately if you find yourself constantly being triggered both mentally and emotionally.

Chapter 2:
Accepting Depression

Looking at the title one would only wonder: Accepting depression, you try! Not so easy if you live it each day. If you battle all other related issues that come with having depression some of our lists can go on for the length of your arm. Others get lucky maybe and only have a few symptoms of depression. To us, those who have the arm length, it will always be a constant battle of strength and weakness. It's going to be a battle of survival for most. There will be ones who constantly fall down, but get right back up to fight and move forward with their life.

Always have in the back of your mind that you need to remember… this process might be slow but every step you take is a step towards becoming whole again. I wish I had someone to tell me to… wake up with fire in your soul with a beautiful vision in your mind. Changing your thought process will be hard! Setbacks will be there from time to time. Your belief means everything. We only have one life at this. I and you reading this need to stand tall, speak loudly, be bold more importantly, be the person you were born to be.

Sometimes taking even as much as a baby step is the hardest day we sometimes have; putting one foot in front of the other is not… not that easy. Some of us manage to pull ourselves together and go through another day of mental anguish that no one ever sees. I am not sure even at my age if I have ever come across anyone that says they have or have had depression. We find out for many when time has come and it's already too late to help even if we wanted to. Depression, if given the power, can extremely change the strongest person to be the weakest.

As I grew older I was hoping for wiser at the same time, but those don't always come hand in hand. The paths I chose to follow had a bearing on my depression for sure. But when you are young and you think you know all and you convince yourself you can, we sometimes make that last step on that path and figure out it only made things worse. If only we could turn back the clock to that very instance we made the wrong choice. Only if we could I don't think I would make the same mistakes in life. The mistakes are neither of my children nor my grandchildren, but of the incidents in between. Sometimes when you strive and leave someone behind in that journey, the prices of doing so could be your life-changing moment you have feared for so long.

There are many reasons why we struggle with things in our lives, some good and of course the dreaded ones. Our intentions are never to have things end in that destructive manner. Our thoughts and admirations get the best of us. As human nature is, we tend to just run with it.

In the years past I have always regretted trusting the wrong people, believing in their words. I forever ignored their actions which led me to believe their loyalty meant nothing. Lesson: they didn't have loyalty towards me as I did them. This happened more times than I could count. Learn early to let these people who drain you go to the curb and don't look back. It will serve you no purpose if you do. Only more heartaches. Not everyone in your life is meant to stay.

Walking through my life has taught me to act tough... hide my pains at any cost, never showing my heartbreak. Growing up I creakily learned that I would be forever by myself. I still feel unwanted by the entire family. My family has had over hundreds of gatherings and I never to this day ever got an invitation. No one ever felt my absence. No one ever noticed my silence. I have forever and still think someday that I am not important. Remember that you are... for you.

Finding a way to calmness and patience in your life. Anything outside that box, leave it you no longer have the capacity to deal with their flaws. I cannot remember how many times I have been so emotionally exhausted. I still stood up to hide my pain; I moved forward always with intense pain. At times I really thought I was coming to the end of my life. I cannot lie and say yeah it has not come across my mind a thousand times. Back then I was barely serving my own life.

How many times have you been close to giving up? How many nights do you sit there and think it is all over? You are still here and you have been through many storms where you thought you would drown. But through your pain and that feels endless you are still here; you are still standing where you need to be. With each new step you gain more strength and carry that with you knowing you are wanting to live in the moment. The next time something or someone steps in your path that tries to break you, always remember you have already survived much worse. You need to keep moving forward; you are not done living yet!

I was told for over a decade that I had to stop looking so bummed out, stop looking like you just lost your best friend. In a great many ways, unannounced to the person telling me to change, it made things go deeper inside me. It began to make me feel as I was getting older I wasn't normal. I would look at my siblings and see no pain in their eyes, no discomfort of who they are supposed to be. I watched my friends grow and grow strong as I stayed behind closed behind the wall I was building. I started my wall at only the tender age of eight.

But by the time I hit twelve years I blocked everything out of my mind. I literally had no memory before my eleventh birthday. Over the years, as I have listened to friends reminisce about childhood, I could not participate. That thought grew to fear, and that fear started to change who I was. I suddenly felt myself being sadder for longer periods. Being young, I was shunned; it led to deeper depression and heartache. Being young with no direction and no help, I placed myself around a very high wall.

I never had the love the other kids received hugs, kisses, the "I love you!" I wished every single day. But my parents only paid attention to me if I was in trouble. They assumed I was tough. I didn't need that for whatever fucken reason. That constant betrayal from my parents and family definitely made me a hardened person at my young age. Even thinking of what I am going to say next makes me cry; it makes me feel like, holy fuck, you made it even after all those painful years beforehand.

By now you are wondering, well how do we accept depression? Well, it all depends on each one of you and in which way it has encompassed your lives. Maybe you haven't felt that deep sensation knowing what was the trigger in the first place? Are you thinking, do we really know? I do believe we do to some extent. It's about you taking the time to put yourself back being involved versus being hidden in the back corner where no one can see you. Remember how you felt; remember how you stood up over that trauma see how it makes you feel now. I believe once you find and pinpoint that exact time you are more willing to go forward with dealing with the disease than you were yesterday.

In all my years I have not known a soul who ever heard my story. No one ever heard my painful cries; I needed help yet no one reached out. No one noticed me and I always stood in silence. I always stood alone. I can say with certainty that they didn't even notice me as part of this family. I was labeled young by my mom's side of the family. Hell no forgiveness whatsoever in that family. I was labeled young as a thief. Exactly where I have been for the last forty-four years.

Finding new ways might depend on learning from others, listening to the harshness of reality. I got really good at hiding my emotions. I am at a point in my life where I don't even care anymore, because I know deep down I am a good person. The sad thing is I cannot force people to see it. I am to the point where I don't fucken care what people think of me! I am ok with people having different opinions of me. I have always been misunderstood. Why change things now in my life?

I always walked alone, not because I wanted to but because I learned very young what betrayals taught me. For me it was safer to be alone than to stay with someone who only pretends to love you, only pretends to be loyal. A quiet heart gives me more comfort than doubts. I will never beg for forgiveness. No one ever gave me that luxury, not even family.

I no longer have the energy to explain my side of the story, especially when they think otherwise. Now is the time I finally do me! Well, that is hard to do for sure, but every day I will step forward and try. Throughout my life I have fought many hard battles that no one sees. I have carried the burden no one knows about. I always showed up for the people I loved until they loved me no more. Got ghosted by my own family.

I have always felt exhausted emotionally, physically and mentally but each time someone needed me I was there. I have given my last shirt to help people. Mentally some days I have been so tired, but each day I moved forward because people needed me and they depended on me. I never had the luxury of breaking down. I think I have gone through more so I can survive this. I cry every day in my shower, I wipe my tears away, get dressed, then walk out like I was okay!

I am fifty-four years old and it's been a journey of many hardships, broken hearts, lost loved ones, divorce, raising children. And I just figured out the onset of my depression. I was not looking for it at the time. To be honest I had put that all in the very back of my mind and left it there to rot. But this one day it all came rushing back to me; it felt so real at the moment in time. It was so overwhelming I was in bed for the next six days just crying my eyes out.

I seriously felt like I was losing my total inner self my self-worth, who I thought I was. Then I saw that finally these were the reasons my heart got cold. My emotions stayed hindered. They stayed so tucked away that I had not done therapy. They would have been left there for the rest of my life. At least that is what I was telling myself. Easier to accept. To this very day, even ten years later, that day haunts me right to my core.

People say when you are dying your life flashes before you. This was that experience the heartbreak, the dire moments of being molested, the memories of being raped over and over again. This was the third time in my life that I had to submit to my emotional breakdown because I mentally lost it. I felt bad for my kids. I hurt even more when I couldn't even pick up my grandson the only person who loved me unconditionally. With days of crying and days of sadness I finally came back. I came back because of my grandson. Oh, I love him to the moon and back and all the stars in the world.

Do you believe that somewhere in your childhood you experienced a horrific or traumatic event? If you have had feelings of being lost, uncontrollable bouts of crying, wanting to be left alone most every time, choosing to be alone throughout life then you can say you suffer from depression. It is better to accept something, even though it is not a positive outcome, because you can turn it into your saving grace. You will find once you accept life for what it is, it is easier to handle. Laugh my ass off, right? Yeah, I would say so too.

But one thing is true regardless of everything falling around you: you have to take control first. If you don't as it did to me and many others before me it will take control of your life; it will change the comfort and normality of your life until you decide you are in control. Please don't give up. Sometimes it is so dark that you cannot see any relief before you. There is definitely more to life still waiting for you to discover. I know more than anybody how much your heart hurts right now.

I know that feeling you are having right now "like you will never get better"? There will still be much more laughter you haven't heard yet, people and places you haven't seen or met. There will be people who will love you in ways you could never imagine. There will be moments coming that will make you feel loved again. As hard as it may be to picture them now, you are not done; this isn't the end of your story. This wasn't mine. I kept going to find the version of who I wanted to be maybe smile again without forcing it. Hope for a better future and hope that your life starts to make sense. You are needed here; you and your life matter more than you know.

No, life does not come with a manual nor does it come with direction in which to live life. OK sure, you can purchase 1,001 books on how to. But not one can know how to kick depression's ass. You will find thousands of journals and manifestos explaining depression, but I truly bet not one person who wrote them actually suffers from depression. Always easier said than done. I am afraid, and unless you personally walk in someone else's shoes you will never know. I would never want to walk in a soldier's shoes after a war. Nor would one of them want to be me and live through being molested, raped and beaten. So which is better? But remember you are NOT the only one to be going through it. You are not alone. Yes, having depression does not make doing anything easy, to say the least. In actual fact it becomes ten times harder to deal with when you have depression.

The biggest misconception of depression is everyone hides the fact they have been diagnosed with it. I, for many, many years, did not accept I had it whatsoever. Most always just said, "you just went through this or that, give it time." Not one, even since I was a young child, would admit or say I had depression. So for the most part I went most of my life without treatment. Not having that made my life extremely harder to deal with and accept, causing me to go through relationships that would just fail. Then I felt worse because I failed once again!!!

No, it didn't get any easier as I grew older. My depression worsened; then, because of some traumatic events, not only did I have depression but PTSD to accompany it. If you find depression is hard, this is a whole new ball game with PTSD it really messes with your mind. The nightmares and the struggles with life are all harder. Waking up each day to deal with it, my attitude was "Fuck off." But the reality was I had to get my ass out of bed; I had to get on with life.

Because I was in a mentally disturbed life, I did not make any good choices well, the exception of my children, of course. But they suffered many hard days with me. As a young mom I had extremely hard days, and to be honest it was hard to be completely there when your own mind and body are so screwed up. The longer I went on with life not treating my depression, life got real hard. You don't make good decisions when your mind is not in a good state. Fears and emotions untreated always take control. You will lose that battle every time until you finally decide to kick depression's ass. I will do my best to never lose hope no matter how heavy the pain gets me down.

The hardest thing to do as a child, even as an adult, is to keep trying to show up no matter what. I remember no matter how I felt, you gotta do this sad: continue working with a broken heart. I was grieving; I did it grieving, mostly I was always doing it tired. Learning that life doesn't care, it doesn't wait for anyone you just remember to take that step forward.

The amount of times I have been let down is completely astonishing and definitely not in a good way. I have been hurt a thousand times, but I still love. Some days I believe I run just on pure willpower. No matter how hard my days got, I can say some were a holy fuck day. I always got up and smiled. I will forever push forward to keep believing that better days are ahead.

It will always come down to you your inner you and your future you taking control that you want life different. You need to have that talk with yourself that you will not let it take over your life nor let it control you living your life. I found that the hardest day of my life. This will be something you always have to do; you will always have to keep picking yourself up off the depression bus and say, "Not today, not this time!" Even after accepting my life-changing issues I will forever have, I keep telling myself to get up! Move forward and let it go!

Yes, I bet you are thinking "easier said than done." Yes, it is each and every time sometimes it is easy, others, well, it will take all the inner energy you have inside you to let go and move on. It is not a matter of self-blaming or blaming someone for pushing you in a direction of losing control. It's now about taking control.

After I finally accepted that I was suffering horrible depression and PTSD, I decided to seek help. I did so with medication I have been on it for over ten years now. Luckily, I suffer no ill side effects from the medication. Well, I have one, and it will happen to anyone having to take medication for depression: pretty much no matter what you take, your libido will suffer. You seem not to have extreme or naughty urges. Believe me, in all sense it is still very much there. You just need to work at things a little harder, tell your significant other to add some foreplay. You will adapt over time and you will find other new ways to build up that fun you may need in the bedroom. Whatever you do, don't believe for one second it is gone for good. Remember we are all human and urges will most definitely come when you are ready.

It is way more important to make sure you are happy in your life. If your life is disorganized then your inner self-destruction is still there. There are a great many kinds of medication you can take. If one doesn't work, try another. It's important for your life to finally take control. Some people just don't understand how much strength it takes to pull yourself out of a dark place mentally. I am far from perfect and I've never claimed to be. My heart overbeats, it overthinks, my mind did have doubts, and my emotions were absolutely hard to tame.

I have certainly made my fair share of mistakes. I've carried pain like no other, my scars from battles no one ever sees. This also gave me strength. I have a soul now that refuses to quit. The constant being silent was wrong; explaining was wrong; crying was wrong; being weak was my downfall. These days people still say what you have done wrong inside while praising you for doing something right.

Everyone needs time to breathe. That being said… take a long deep breath and focus on you. Find a place you can gravitate to that brings you peace. Find a place in your mind where you can stand still and regroup. Your inner peace is as important as anything else. Taking a step back isn't about escaping the problems but rather about finding the clarity and strength to face them head on.

Remember you can always cry not because something happened, but simply for being you. The war we have inside our own heads never slows down. We feel everything too deeply in our world. People's values have become indifferent. Showing up when I've got nothing left to give I still cry because I carry too much in my silence. The night sees my heartache; my pillow knows my truths. My silence is the only one that never asks me to explain my pain. When someone realizes I haven't slept, they don't understand what it is like when I can't just stop thinking and remembering and fighting the constant pain.

Something that took me a while to learn was that my most dangerous anger is built up. Even people with a good heart I have just been played too many times for being there for people who only took advantage of my kindness. Never let someone change who you are into what they need. Always remember to be you believe me, this will be tested over and over again. Be you, walk straight and start a new day and walk your way to some peace.

As I have walked through life I warrant a smile, but behind that smile lies a quietly unraveling. With luck the cracks are never seen as I mastered the art young at hiding them. Some days it is easier to laugh on cue; I always say I am OK! Since I was young it became part of my script that I have memorized. I cannot explain how many times, while carrying the heaviest of things, I never speak of them.

One day the truth will come to light: that you are not breaking you can say you are not OK, that you are breaking. You don't need to say it in a loud voice everyone will hear or notice, but in a quieter, invisible moment only you can see. Healing isn't always becoming someone new. It is finally facing what you never wanted to feel.

By grieving what you pretend, it need not hurt you. You need to finally let go of the old version of you. Do not hold it in; let it out. Healing will always be messy you will fall and you will cry for your rage, exhaustion, silence; this will also become your power. There will be that moment you decide to stop running from all your pain. One day you will remember who you were before the world tore you apart.

You never need to be loud to become brave; you simply just need to keep going. Standing tall and believing in yourself is the most important. Losing yourself never meant you are weak; it just meant you were drowning under the pressure of the weight you carry on your shoulders. It means stop bending until it breaks you, stop giving until you become empty. There is no need to keep proving your worth.

Sometimes things will feel as though those memories and that pain are gone forever. One day you will bury things and finally feel safe enough to come back to wanting to be you. My goodness, on the amount of times people asked me, "Are you not going to tell your side of the story?" Why the fuck should I? To this very day I have been challenged a few dozen times over.

Telling my side of the story never mattered when I already could see what was said about me they made me into this liar. In people's eyes I was made to be this ugly person they were making me out to be. Truth is I was never that person they said I was. I was finally so tired of fighting that I gave up caring.

Holy fuck talk about people bashing me. My exes did unbelievable damage on top of my two girls. I still fight battles I should not be fighting. I am fighting ghosts; the person they made me out to be was beyond horrific, beyond comprehension. I was at a loss for words most of the time. I just got so tired of fighting, as she said.

Fighting took way too much of my mental and physical health; I stayed unhealthy physically for years well, actually for a few decades. My father's favourite thing was to give me a hard time about my weight. Now I give him a hard time. Damn turned fifty and gained like thirty pounds. I have to say being heavier made me feel healthier.

Unfortunately, I was way too young when my trauma started and as much as I wished and dreamed of things changing, it never happened for me. Life honestly does change when you finally want it to. If you don't want it, then it won't happen. When you want it you must grab hold of it and accept the change to happen.

I could probably write a few books just on trying to kick depression's fucken ass. Unfortunately, depression is lifelong. But it doesn't have to be that hard anymore. It doesn't mean you need to carry the burden of the world on your shoulders. Life isn't meant to be easy, but it is also not meant to be this hard. This change comes from you first. Remember I am right beside you holding your hand.

These past three weeks have been more than my heart and body could handle. I fell into a selfish state of self-depression. For days I tried to grab him with my emotions, my thoughts, my feelings but it didn't work. I feel I lost weight, sleep physically and emotionally exhausted. I stood alone dealing with the fact I found my amazing boss deceased.

I got to work about 6:45, the freezer wasn't working so I asked the other employee to go wake her up. She came and said she couldn't get in her room so I went to go through the back door. This door led into her room. My heart told me to take a deep breath. I opened the door and I looked straight forward to the other door hoping something was against it.

My beautiful boss lay there naked, cold and lifeless. I called, of course, knowing they were not going to be there quickly as I stated, she was already gone. He felt the same, but her color and her stillness said otherwise. I knew in my heart her soul may be gone, but I grabbed a blanket off her bed and covered her up.

I then hung my phone up, sat down beside her and talked. I talked about being sorry if I had caused her heartache. I said I was sad it wasn't time yet I had just started to get to know her. I was loving working for her, doing her markets oh boy those were so much fun. It was amazing for my wellbeing. She was such a beautiful soul. Much light will be lost from her being gone. As I talked and finally said, "You can go," I saw imprints in the blanket like someone was pushing themselves up. I felt then she left I seriously felt her final goodbye. The saddest thing is that her mother died two weeks prior. Oh, I will miss her. I had a bad day once and she walked over and gave me such a huge hug I cried. I had never felt an honest, true "I love you" hug. That she had me in her arms actually caring, loving me even for that moment oh, I will miss her forever.

Sitting with someone who is deceased is not an easy thing to handle. If you have to deal with that in your life, take that opportunity to say your goodbye, to tell them it is ok to go. You have that one last chance for no regrets. Never have regrets suffering from depression, that is a battle I do not know how to handle. Hopefully you will if that happens.

Unfortunately, in doing that sitting with a beautiful friend that has passed also leaves images that are extremely hard to forget and release from your memory and eyes. For almost three weeks when I would look down at the floor or ground I would see my beautiful friend laying there cold, no movement, no breathing. I see myself next to her. It buries itself in the deepest part of my memory, my feelings and mentally I just couldn't let go.

The few weeks after that just snowballed; my anger showed itself and I literally had to walk away. But the anger I have felt about a certain person still drives my anger. All I truly want to do is ouch the living fuck out of her even today. Disgusted when I see her name, when I hear her name being mentioned in a conversation. I have a hatred that I seriously need to release.

Yes, I still have trouble even writing, but the writing also fuels the extreme emotions I fester. It is yes still hard. It was harder because at the same time, dealing with her death, another friend's life was in the balance of losing her life. My dear friend was losing her battle with a brain tumour. As a friend I feel anger towards her parents and, yeah, a little towards the man who loved her.

It is not okay to choose your feelings over the wishes of any loved one. My friend I knew over fourteen years and I always knew she had the tumour in her brain. She always stated her true beliefs in DNR she didn't want to live in a disabled life, a life where she could not be herself. Damn this wonderful human was so talented, a spirit like no other and a love like no one could give. Her parents didn't do as her wish was.

For eight grueling months she struggled not being herself. You see, women when we have a stroke we often have paralysis on the right side. Jo was an amazing artist, all around a beautiful woman who got robbed. Out of selfishness only. The sad thing was that it didn't faze them. It was so wrong. When I went to see her for her wedding days I never saw so much pain in someone's eyes as I did that day. Oh fuck for the last three weeks…

Every second of every single day I struggled opening up Facebook, each time wondering if today I would see my friend's passing. Each day my anxiety went through the roof. Day in and day out it stayed the same. Until yesterday they finally moved her to palliative care. Until this morning my anxiety and pain flooded my life.

Today, as I hit the page to open, I see she had passed at 10:30 this morning. My heart felt relief, it suddenly felt at peace. I suddenly felt she was no longer in pain and she could be that beautiful artist once again. Heaven has gained amazing angels. I will forever miss them both. Not everyone gets to be remembered in my life, that's for sure.

Remember we all have a few bad days, and we will continue to. It comes down to how you deal with it in the end. Unfortunately, there will also be times where it causes more emotional stress. Just remember you need to take care of you too. If you are not eating, at least eat some crackers. That's my bad habit not eating it could become dangerous.

It is always okay if you cannot handle a day or a family gathering. Maybe you just need to be with you. Remember there are people who will support you, who will grab your hand and say, "I got you." That is the friend to keep. Grief and heartbreak are very difficult to deal with, to overcome, to handle, and then move on.

I have been racking my head trying hard to figure out how I am going to handle a celebration of life. When I found my boss deceased, a friend went through the roof with dramatics dramatics that set me into anger. The longer the day went on, the angrier I got. Honestly, I have not let that feeling quit yet. My blood is still boiling, and yet I know I should just let it go.

I have had a hundred reasons to forgive and move on, but the underlying principle stands in my way. What angered me was her calling me and telling me I had to live with the fact that her and me fighting bothered her. I apologized for my behaviour. But she will never change her narcissistic tendencies.

Forgiving and forgetting are two separate things, and both need to be addressed appropriately. I have forgiven way too much in my life, even after people have hurt me over and over again throughout my life. Some forgiving will serve its purpose, and some will not. That depends on your own personal journey. I suppose I will see what kind of journey I take at the celebration of life for my first friend.

Chapter 3:
Moving Forward

Moving forward is it really that easy? Most would say no. I can say, although it's been a very hard road at times, giving up is not in my vocabulary. Should it be? No, it shouldn't. If it is, then it just shows you never yelled loud enough or to the right person. Yes, it may take a bit of time to find that right person to help you, guide you, and lead you. But you will find that person. You first have to allow yourself to want to find the person who is supposed to help you through this. We are never meant to be alone, no matter the circumstances before us.

For some of us, moving forward is not going to be easy. For some, we may have to get up on our own a few times before we accomplish our goals of suppressing our depression. I did not get it the first time, nor the second or third. I finally gave up counting the times I got up on my own after I had fallen. But each time I had fallen, I got back up regardless of having someone or no one. The more I watched people succumb to this dreadful disease, the more it made me want to strive not to end up losing my battle on living life. Life may not be full of all the excitement one may be looking for, but happiness must first come from you.

Is moving forward the best for everyone? I would have to say it is the best for you. It doesn't matter if it makes it easier for the loved ones around you. Stop trying to please them and do it for yourself first. Yes, sitting there, you are thinking, "Yeah, easier said than done!" I thought those same words each and every time I had to get back up on my feet. At some point, you need to decide if you want to control it or have it control you.

Over the years, I have mastered the art of holding myself together in public. It became second nature to act and look the part of being fine. Through my entire life and my journey of finding myself, I learned that saying "I am fine," two simple words, can feel so true but only at times. In silence, no one ever sees my pain; they certainly cannot see the heavy burden that I carry.

My depression controlled my life for well over a decade before I chose to rethink the state in which I was presently living. After so long of being in a depressive state, it was one of the hardest things in my life I had to overcome. No, I still haven't overcome depression, but at least now I can live without it controlling me as much. Unfortunately, depression isn't something we can just take a pill for and it's gone. Don't we wish it was that easy? People surely would be a great deal happier if that were the case. But you can move forward when you look at it in a different light. We are all born with free will, and that free will gives you your option of moving forward, taking a different stride in the direction you were once going. You must take a personal stand against depression. It is only a game our body is trying to play. It's time to strike back with harder force and determination.

Over the last few days, I found myself falling into a deep depression, and believe me, it was coming at a much faster rate this time. I cried for a few days and realized it's not necessary for it to win this time. Yes, I am heartbroken like never in my life. My three grandbabies were moving, and with my oldest grandbaby, he and I have an unbelievable relationship. Two years ago, I suffered a major manic depressive episode, and it caused a chain reaction PTSD and depression that short-circuited and now I suffer from fibromyalgia. For weeks I was so sick I could not walk from bed to bathroom.

Sleeping without being in pain was another story. But through it all, my grandson stayed right by me. He wanted to sleep next to me. Each night, if I was sweating, he took off the blanket, and when I was cold, he did the reverse. When it came time to see the doctor, he would sit on his bum and go down the stairs right next to me, offering his hand to help me walk the few steps to the car. He is always my reason to get up and fight. He is my reason to win each and every battle.

We all may not be blessed with such a beautiful reason to live, but looking deep inside of your inner self, there are already ten reasons to move forward:

1. The best and most important is you.

2. Mental health.

3. Emotional well-being.

4. Physical health your body deserves care and healing.

5. Peace of mind finding calm within yourself.

6. Strength to face tomorrow, even when today feels unbearable.

7. The chance to create memories that have not yet been written.

8. The love you give and the love you are yet to receive.

9. The dreams and goals you still hold inside of you.

10. Hope because without it, there is no reason to keep going.

There is one important reason why most of us who suffer from depression or PTSD keep how we feel and the thoughts we think to ourselves for more than one reason or another. I know, as I have become a mom and now a grandma, no one can fix what they don't know is broken. Although yes, we are not broken, we still have parts that are breaking and need mending. I am one of the most guilty ones for not coming forward in my adult life. I tried when I was a kid maybe not in the correct way but nonetheless tried to act out so someone would listen. Maybe I was hoping as a child they could read my mind and stop the destruction that was beginning to take my innocence as a child, then my teens, and straight on into adulthood.

Moving forward takes passion, determination, willpower, and strength. We all have these; maybe we just haven't found them quite yet. Remember they are there you just need to find them. The first time I took a foot forward was, believe it or not, after I had read *The Secret*. That small little book opened my eyes to a different direction in which I was seeking answers. I realized I had lost the willpower to love myself first; then I could love life and anything around my life.

Although I truly knew at a young age I suffered from being depressed, I would never say a word to anyone after a while. I never showed my anger, frustration, hurt, or sadness. I thought to get through life I had to pretend to move forward and just keep my little secret of being so internally and emotionally sad to myself. Most of my life I have not been emotionally happy, and it has been a very hard road at times. But each day I put one foot in front of the other and move. No, of course I don't always want to, but life kinda kicks your ass and you need to. Giving in slowly leads to giving up, and that should not be an answer.

Over the years, I have learned that when things are a blur and you're about to give up, and you also realize that you randomly break down, this is when you begin to realize a lot of things while you cry. Owning those realizations is always a part of the healing process. Remember: it is never okay for someone to hurt you in any way. I learned early that I would rather be hated for who I truly am than to be loved or adored for someone I am not. If your love is based on lies, it will never flourish. It is not meant to be. It is far better to be who you are, with no regrets about who you want to be. You need to believe in yourself.

I noticed through my journey that you don't want to be embarrassed by the false side of you. People do not change who you are to suit other people in your life. You certainly don't have to love everyone. Live by "what you see is what you get," and you will not change to suit them anymore.

Over our lifetime, we have all done bad things, and with growing certainty we make more bad and poor decisions. You will grow, you will learn, and you will always remember to be true to yourself. Most times, I have to say, I smile to pretend I am happy. In doing so, it has spared me a thousand conversations I didn't want to have. I have let people believe in the illusion they already see me as.

For me, explaining the truth if ever asked I no longer have it in me. Explaining the truth will always require more strength I no longer have for them. I learned most people don't want the truth; comfort is the only simplicity they want. The utter mess that lives inside my heart, deep inside my chest, behind my smile, has always been my armor.

The storms you walk through don't mean you have to trust anyone. They will never see the burden and pain you carry. I expect you are a bit like me you hide your emotional and mental well-being. Remember, it is okay to break down sometimes. Let that mask of smiles fall. Maybe today someone will see behind the walls you have built. Just one person can believe in you enough to lighten your heavy load. Sometimes, maybe this time, it will give you the strength to move forward instead of taking you down.

It never fails when the moment you get quiet, suddenly they care… nah. The only thing they seem to miss is my energy, only to constantly use me when they need me and in the end still leave me behind. Still left with the silence and my pain. Then they had the gall to say I was cold. I wasn't cold I was just empty. The countless days I wished upon a star that someone would heal me, that they would just hold me... no one ever did, nor did they ever love me. No one has a clue who I really am.

I cannot imagine the pain or hell you are presently going through, the prices you have to pay, the walls you've learned to build. Every bit of person you are is who I once was. I was afraid. I was lonely. I was broken just like you. I am here to help you. You can get through this. You can survive and finally become stronger. Walk with the knowledge that you can seriously do this. You've got this. I believe in you.

As hard as it may seem on those stormy days, remember to love those who remember you. Challenges will always cross your path, balancing your energy and self-worth. I was never smart enough when I was younger to stop wasting time on people who constantly drained me. Holy, the amount of friends I have lost along my path. They never stuck around when I needed them the most. Be alert to the fake, hollow promises. Focus on the empty smiles. Protect your energy. Protect your inner peace.

My value was never measured by how many friends I had or how many clung to using me. I measured it by the quality of those who stayed by my side. As you move through life, people will forget you, as you will forget them. The loss of losing the untrue, the unfaithful ones will forever be your gain. As you grow and heal, keep your circle small.

Keep your circle honest and true. Always guard your heart and keep your mental mind sharp. Respect is only earned by balance and trust. Remember to cherish those true connections you make through your life. Let go of the ones who serve you no purpose in your life. I have learned that you can say goodbye to those loved ones as quickly as they appeared in your life.

I am sure if you are reading this you are on the path of trying to figure out, or looking for the explanation of, heartache. There are so many ways our hearts can break love, loss, emotional and mental heartbreak. To be honest, I never wanted to be loved. My heart broke for years trying to find someone. My heart was already broken, not healed; it was emotionally done. No matter how hard I tried, it just wasn't possible not for me anymore.

Trying to find a person able to accept you for who you really are. Finding a person to just love you and want nothing but the world for you. My heart was never ready to be loved. It was, and is still, broken. I spend most of the day alone. I am happy being by myself even today. I don't have to put energy into people. Yes, I do try every now and then. I did well twice. I tried to make a community and that backfired. I lost everything that made my space feel like home.

Feeling at home... well, fuck, that doesn't happen often if at all. I spent most of my entire life feeling unsettled. The emotional toll it took on me year after year... but I found that place when I wasn't even looking. Because I let my guard down, I got seriously screwed lost my job, my home, my feeling of safety. Out of anger, and only equipped with half the knowledge, I was immediately kicked out. My peace of mind, my emotional and physical state sent me on a whirlwind path. How it was done was so extremely wrong.

When bad people or outright assholes like my old landlords use their power to make good people homeless, something should be done. You would think especially in today's world... but no. I live somewhere I totally despise, certainly not at all good for my depression. Trying to explain the heartache and heartbreak of just wanting to be loved, knowing in your heart you are not.

Finding love was impossible for me. It was impossible to find someone to accept me for who I was emotionally, physically, and mentally broken. Shit, I was seriously broken long before I was seventeen. How sad it is to write or for someone to read. Experiencing life back in my day certainly wasn't easy. Man, the memories wishing to forget them. But I suppose they are what made me who I am. Who I want to become. Every day is a new learning day, a new realization of your desire for more.

Since I could remember, I had one wish and one wish only: just one person would love me. Just one. One day it's going to be the last day your last phone call to your mom, the last time you smelt a rose, the last day you felt at peace. We all will have that last day. Having regrets is hard to live with. They do not go away. Say what you need to say to have your peace.

Time to say your peace, or to get your peace, will soon be unreachable. Time will disappear. Then one day it will become an old memory. You will hear your last song. There has been a new man who has woken up from his versions of moving on. Every time I listen to him, I feel that I want to reach out and grab him and just say… I understand. I got you. I love his music. ❤

Listening to his songs has been refreshing while suffering from depression. It has felt like, a few times listening, that holy I get it. I understand what these lyrics mean. Learning is growing, and growing soon becomes knowledge to put one step in front of the other even if you are not ready. Shit, I have never been ready. No better time than now.

As I have reflected on my life, I have noticed most of my mistakes were just loving the wrong people but also trusting them. These people had convinced me at that time to trust them, to believe in them. They are the very ones who constantly caused me the most pain. My loyalty to people, even my family, were the first to leave or never showed when I really needed them. I learned to stand alone. Sometimes that is the best for me.

Oh believe me, I had a thousand arguments with myself. I always tried to believe the best in people, yet in the back of my mind I was ready for the disappointment the total ignorance of family. So many times I got to witness firsthand their actions. I am not sure, even at 54, can I say I ever witnessed any family member believe in me or even just say, "I love you." I think I am the only niece or nephew who has never been told they were loved.

I felt that for decades. Then my grandmother was passing. My sister looks at me in the room and with extreme discussion with me tells me to say goodbye, and while you're at it, apologize. I was set back I mean really. She left and I said my goodbyes. I also stated reasons I did things, but yet no one asked. My grandmother believed I called the police on her neighbor because he sold pot. Like seriously I was a pot smoker, a heavy one, a true pothead. Why would I?

As I talked with my grandmother, she had tears running down the left side of her cheek. Yes, I do believe she heard me. I believe she finally understood some of my pain. My grandmother dying just added to my depression by a thousand times no thanks to my sister.

I will never be able to explain how destroyed emotionally, mentally, and physically I broke. I cried for days. I was lost physically. I couldn't even stand up, and being emotionally exhausted left me without an appetite for six days. My mind, my body was in complete and utter chaos. My grandson looked at me, lost. His expression almost killed me. He crawled up, wrapped his little arms around me, and held me so tight. I felt my life would be okay.

When people are behind closed doors, they will always compete, they will gossip, and they will continue to be fake. When I was young, I was under the false belief that all people were good. Pain taught me one important thing: always read between the lines and their disturbing smiles.

At some point in your life, you will learn to watch more and speak less. Sometimes when you share, it falls on deaf ears. They never listen and certainly do not understand. Mistakes are meant to be made, or we would never learn. We are human and we are not perfect. We are meant to make mistakes big ones, small ones, and ones that will certainly embarrass you. Your mistakes will never define you. Your proof that you are searching for is... you are trying. Learning is absolutely growing.

Remember one thing: their opinion will never matter. Their opinion will never fulfill your dreams. Moving forward be true to yourself, be honest, own your mistakes, but learn from those days. Success is certainly not about being perfect or humble. It is about moving forward, never giving up, keeping one step ahead of the other, and moving forward. You got this. I believe in you.

Remember, it is not just you. A ton of people have been through something. They have something that has changed them just as if it was you or me. Never judge a book by its cover. You can never know what demons they are fighting. Reach your hand out, just as you want them to do with you. How many times have you seen no one reach out to you?

Those ones always left you high and dry. How many times did it take you to finally realize you were on your own as usual? Finding out and knowing people are not there for you. I have certainly had many lonely days. It was hard knowing no one was showing up for me, no matter how much I would beg. No one even asked why I needed support. It never fazed a single family member. As the days and years crept forward.

The stress, the emptiness, the feeling of not being loved has still broken me. When I fell apart, the silence, the emotional disconnect everyone was always too busy to help. More so, they just didn't want to help. You need to fix yourself to help yourself. Discovering yourself is the most important part of living. Remind yourself of your own worth. No one has, or will ever have, the power to crush your dreams but you.

I hope telling you my truths helps you feel inspired to do the same with your life. I don't know if life will be good, but the friends you make will help you become the person you want to be. Believe in trust but always keep your mind open.

Notice the ones who want you to suffer, the ones who want to break you. You need to realize that you have been there for everyone. Now realize absolutely no one has been there for you. You will realize, just as I did, that you were never the priority. I realized early that I was only an opinion, I was only ever a pit stop for the ones who pretended to love me who broke me more by showing me how truly they did not love me and how I am never missed.

I always wonder if my family or friends ever thought I was strong enough. I learned I had absolutely no one to talk to growing up well, fuck, even now at my age. Should I be angry? I would absolutely say fuck yes. My high and mighty family who never does wrong!

News alert: you left a family member behind. You let someone suffer. You let them believe they were never, nor are they now, loved. It's so hard I look every day for someone to say something but I know deep down I will never, ever get an apology. I will never, ever be loved by my family. I am okay with that. I am just so done with the pain, I am done feeling unloved, I am done with all my mental problems you all have given me. I suppose I would forgive, as it is the person I am, regardless of the lack of love and emotion from the ones who said they loved me the most.

Some of those mistakes you will regret deeply in that moment, although it felt like the right thing to do. As you walk through life, be the new friend you make along the way. Never change yourself to suit them. That will only lead to more trauma and more pain.

You must be thinking by now either "Wow, she really has suffered like me!" or "Is it just another pretender giving me advice or leading me in a different direction?" I have suffered, and on a daily basis battle my biggest fight each and every day since I was a very young child. From being that very innocent young girl to the mother and grandma I am now, suffering with depression has made me a very strong, independent person who, after years of losing, decided to just get up and fight.

Fighting and continuing to fight is not optional for me. I have grandchildren who adore me and love me unconditionally. They don't know Nana fights with the devil on a daily basis. But I won for them. This time it feels like the worst has happened to me. Yet, on the other hand, it is a good thing for my daughter and her family. The crushing factor to me is my grandson leaves with them. He and I have been through the best and worst together so far. He's always picking me up on a bad day. He's my savior and saving grace. All my grandkids are a saving grace.

For over three years I have gotten to see him grow and learn and be by his Nana. Now suddenly he won't be my day. My normal life for so long has to change, and in a huge way. Fear sets in. Emotions will run fast and far over the next month. Things I thought I could do because of him will have to change. My strength, my partner in growing, is leaving my side and oh yeah, this mom/grandma is scared shitless.

Being scared moving forward is also a good thing. I have cried for days and I am very sure I will continue to cry, but I will remind myself it's for the better good of her family. It's her life and not about mine. After I cried really hard for a few days, I had to look in the mirror and decide: "Are you going to fall down or are you going to pick yourself back up?" That brought me to this very moment. I decided to get up and kick its ass this time harder and better than I have ever done. This time, this depressive episode will not get the better of me. I have chosen after many years to share my story. Even if it never gets published! I move forward with my grandbabies. I need them as much as they need me. I am not that old yet, so I don't need a walker.

An old memory way back when I was in grade 8/9 English with Mrs. Beetle. She wanted so much for me to write then. She nagged me constantly to write. I can remember her so angry with me as I kept telling her, "That will not get me anywhere in life, writing on emotions." And look here I am, writing about not only emotions but deadly life-threatening diseases I get to contend with each and every day of my life. I used my writing back then in class to release the sadness I felt, the emotions I didn't know how to deal with or express. She thought I had a gift to say it as it is. And yeah, people, it is hard but that doesn't mean you have to quit.

Moving forward is looking forward to the best of what life can bring you. You may stumble a bit, but who doesn't? We all do once in a while. Take every step as if it were your first. Try something new if the last thing you tried didn't work for you. As hard as it is… try, try again. Get up and do it again. One day you will find the peace in yourself you are looking for. It's not about what people want us to be it's about who and what you want to be. No one is perfect, and we are all here for a purpose in life, as hard as it may seem.

In my lifetime, I have seen the best come down with this disease. It is a major killer of many good people each year. The last being Robin Williams what a great inspiration to so many, young and old. He brought so much laughter, light, and belief to all who watched him in movies and in the personal lives he touched. I will never forget the joy and admiration my uncle had when he told me he received a personalized book *Jumanji*, which read: *"To Gary Williams from Robert Williams."* No relation to one another, but

47

my uncle thought it was the best thing ever to receive in his life. My uncle was a grip in the movies he did not have a part in. So very touching, and a humble thing from the heart to do.

On and off since his death, I have bounced around the idea only in my head to tell my story. Then I looked around and saw lots of people telling their stories. But all seemed to cite authors, doctors, etc. This is not going to cite things unless it happened personally to me. There is no book out there that can change our thoughts, our depression, or the uneven state we live in and through. But I do believe words are stronger when they come from true stories, true emotions, and life events that brought us to this place. Life is not about how many doctors you have they have no bearing on my life or my depression. I do. And I want you to realize you are the best person to make yourself stand up and change the direction in which you handle this fucked-up shit.

Do you have the thought that maybe you can move forward with therapy? Excellent thinking in the right direction, maybe for some! You need to find the right person, and that is not, in any way, an easy thing to do depending on where you live. For children seeking help, that is a much harder task, I think personally, and it left me always having a hatred for child psychologists. Unfortunately, when I needed the help as a very young child, it backfired. The psychologist although under confidentiality turned around and told my parents what I had said. That turned into massive fights, arguments, and more personal torment to my emotions. Anything I had said was twisted around to make me look like a liar and to convince me I was wrong to think those thoughts and to have them. When that happened, it taught me how to put my emotions and feelings deep down and never discuss them with anyone again.

Did I always keep those beliefs? I would say they have not changed in me, even still at 44. That damaged me so intensely that it scarred me for the rest of my life. Then, when I was becoming depressed and no one listened, it was chalked up to "acting out" as far as my parents and the psychologist were concerned nothing more. What was already giving me depression became a powerful psychological breakdown before I was the age of nine. By the time I hit pre-teen years, I had already been sexually assaulted for years. I had been abused physically for years.

I had lost the only relationship I cherished with my father. He suddenly stopped looking at me as his little girl, and all his anger began to be directed at me for years to come. I don't think, to this day, my dad ever realized he was doing it. But that wouldn't have changed the outcome. At that point in my father's life, he needed a place or a person to take his frustrations out on, and it just happened to be me. All these issues I had to hide. I had to bury them so deep inside me that they ate away at me each and every day.

Yes, those emotions and feelings from so long ago are still present in my mind. Some come out to haunt me every now and then. But now I see things much differently, and most importantly, I know that even though I gave up hope on one person, I should not have let that stop me from getting help. But it did, and now I just deal with it I rethink things from my past with a more open mind. Our minds are funny. They never forget words, or physical touch, nor do our minds forget pain. As time goes on, you can find a way to deal with the old pain and bring forth a better emotion or well-being to the old way of thinking.

Over the years, I did develop a new way of thinking about seeing a psychologist. I was attending college, working on starting toward a law degree. As suddenly as that journey began, that journey changed just as swiftly. Just as I thought my life was going well I had just gotten engaged that June day in 1999 my boyfriend went off to work. I was sitting, playing a game of crib, and the phone rang. That one phone call altered and changed my life in a downward spiral for the next few years. Not only was I suffering from deep depression, but I was also suddenly going down a volcanic explosion of my mind, losing control. Parts of my mind have never been the same since.

Due to the accident my boyfriend had endured that day, it left me with massive PTSD. I gathered myself back together for what I could at the time being a mother of six and a wife. I suddenly changed from wanting to be a lawyer to wanting to be a psychologist myself. One day, I was attending a class and my teacher asked me to stay behind. He wanted to discuss an issue with me. I tell you, my heart was racing and my stomach was turning. My fear was so deep not only was he my teacher, he was rated the third top psychologist in BC. By the time class ended, I was soaked in sweat. I was white as a ghost, and he knew it.

My teacher got up, locked the doors to class, turned down one set of lights, and walked toward me. I was freaked out like never before. But he sat across from me and quietly said, *"It's okay to let it all out, no matter how far you would like to go back. I am not taking notes. I am not your doctor, and most importantly, I am not here to judge you."*

For the first time in my life and it had been a hard one I heard the words I always wanted to hear: that it was okay. I fell to the ground and sat there and cried and cried. My teacher just calmly sat beside me and said, *"Let it all out. When you do, we will talk."* After several hours of crying, I finally wiped the tears away, got up, and said, *"Now what?"* He looked at me and said, *"One thing at a time. You decide what it is you think you need, and you ask me."*

For the first time, I was at a loss for words. I was scared to say how I felt. The feelings I had when I was a child were rushing back in. I got scared. My face showed him fear and my eyes began to fill with tears. In a quiet voice, he said, *"I have no one to tell any stories you may want to talk about. I have no one to tell your secrets to. It's just the four walls between you and my ears. My hand is only to guide you in the right direction for yourself. And that direction you must figure out when you are ready to do so."*

Since that day my teacher took my hand, I have looked at life differently, and I have sought help sooner rather than later. I have shared with very few the story that changed my life. I have continued, no matter how bad I have felt, to always think of his words to me that day. I never stand up right away. I take my time I take the time I need to work through that emotion first. Then I get up off my ass and put one foot in front of the other. Depression is our worst enemy, and it will fight, and it will be a constant fight, as there is no damn cure for it.

Acceptance is the first step forward, regardless of which step you are taking. This could be your first step in acceptance and your first foot forward. Or, it could possibly be like me, and it's the fiftieth time I've put the same damn foot forward and stepped the same way forward and onward. Today, let it be the first day of a new start. Start kicking depression's ass instead of it laying claim to your beautiful life to be.

Yeah, it is hard. I will admit that. And a few times it almost won with me. Life is worth more than letting it beat you. Believe me, you can have a very happy, full life with lots of people who love you. Guess what? They love you even with the faults you think you may have. Those faults are what make us who we are and who we strive to become. Those faults include depression and all its subcategories: feeling weak, tired, no sense of self-worth, no reason in one's mind to get off your ass and of course, the physical pain our bodies go through.

The physical pain we endure from depression is crucial to our well-being, and it is the most important reason why you must find an outlet of release. As long as my memory serves me, doctors have always sought the prescription route to fix the pain of those suffering from depression. Most have veered away from offering help of any sort other than medication an easy fix to a huge problem that a great many face in real life. I think I lost count after a hundred or so medications that have been offered to me. I am one of the lucky ones. I am highly allergic to sulfa, which takes me out from being able to be a guinea pig with medication. Although, yes, it might have helped me deal with some of the pains I was having, but it wasn't the solution to solve the issue either.

I finally stepped forward with alternate sources of fixing myself. I thought pain from depression was bad. Then I fell into a manic depressive state and my brain gave out sensors and locators, and I ended up with fibromyalgia. If you already suffer from depression and you have not yet reached this level, I advise you with all my heart and soul: stay away from the body fighting back with this. Don't let your depression win. Take control and find a solution to better your health.

There will be, for everyone, successes and failures in trying something new. Get back up and make yourself try another direction to solve your inner issue. When the day finally came that I could walk again without the help of a cane and walker, a friend brought me for a ride up island to take care of and look into property his boss owned. It only took minutes for me to fall in love with the place located right on the river. Beautiful backyard and so much untouched potential in landscaping. I looked at him and mentioned that this place would make tons of money as a B&B during the summer.

A few days later, my friend returned and said, "How about it?"

I replied, "How about what?"

He said, "About the B&B. You up to it?"

What a dream to run a B&B right on the river in one of the best places on the island. I never thought about how much pain my body was still in. It never entered my mind that physically, if I couldn't do this, how the hell was I going to do this? That was the only look on my daughter's face and it was a priceless moment. I jumped at the chance without looking back. My dear friends kept their thoughts to themselves, but my family was not raised that way. A few ideas were thrown around, but in the end, it was still my choice. I chose that day to win.

My option at that time, from the doctors' review of my case, was that I would more than likely be in a wheelchair within a year and that would be for life.

Some days you end up looking at life or taking life for what it is at the time. My amazing summer journey came to an end. It was now back to everyday living. Pain was setting back in, as I had no release anymore nowhere to focus the pain on something else. I was back to living alone in my quiet little apartment. Fall was setting in and the weather was starting to change. The aches and pains were coming back tenfold because of the damp, rainy weather off the coast of Victoria.

When you suffer from depression, it is hard in the winter, especially with the lack of sun for Vitamin D. For the most part, people who suffer will always be in more pain in fall and winter due to lack of sun, lack of energy, and lack of motivation in the cloudy, damp weather. Most people I know who suffer from one form of depression or another are extremely more secluded in the months of fall and winter. I know I am. Going out is the biggest, most feared experience in the winter months. Not to mention, the body aches and pains are more severe in colder, damper weather. More pain means less motivation, less mental thought of wanting to even see your best friend. Isolation is winter's best friend; it has many of us under its control.

You truly need to be adamant about taking vitamins daily in those months when Jack Frost is hanging around. I take Vitamin D, Vitamin B complex, and more veggies and fruit intake as well. Taking them faithfully each day works. You could also take St. John's Wort. Ask your pharmacy as well they are a great help.

In comparison, this depression is first about taking control of it yourself. You need to help you. You need to decide if you are done living in constant hell, loneliness, pain, and unworthy feelings. You are more than that. Believe me, you are. We all have a purpose; we just need to find out what it is meant to be for each of us.

Moving forward might seem like a misconception, but taking these steps forward with your strength, your knowledge, and your better understanding of forgiveness will guide you to a better you a stronger, better you. Move forward if you know now to call out those people who push you down. Tell them firmly: *"You no longer control me. Fuck off."*

Yahoo for you. Say it with me: **Hurrahh!!!.**

I bet that feels really good. Step up more each day and life will keep getting better. Start believing in yourself now. Stand tall you got this. You have the say on who stays and who goes out of your life, remember that. If they make you hurt, the curb is right there. If the curb isn't there, kick them out the fuckin' door. You will have to change directions a few times, I am sure. Life isn't that easy for everyone, but take it in strides and it will lead the way.

I hope your life lets you deal with death a little easier than me. I hope you never have to deal with finding someone deceased. The whole process is long, grueling, and exhausting not to mention the toll on your emotional well-being. If you are a parent and your child passes, please really think about whether you want to look at them after they are gone. That image will never leave your mind. Your eyes will see that image all day and through your dreams even those traumatic daydreams.

There is never a right way or a wrong way when it comes to death. I hope you had better experiences than me. A misconception about death I don't believe you need to attend every memorial service. I believe at times it is better to say goodbye in your own way, in your own time.

Chapter 4:
Never ending Journey

The title of this chapter, *"Never Ending Journey,"* serves almost everyone who suffers from depression. I know from a personal standpoint, as well as having my own never-ending journey. I do believe that if I was given a choice when I was a young child, I would have chosen life without such hardships. I could have gone without as much trauma in my life. Although we cannot get away from life and death, I would have wished for losing fewer important people in my life. Having depression has locked me into a long life of challenges and has certainly made me the person I am today.

Suffering from depression has never been, nor will it ever be, easy. It is a hard, long road in life. Given the right chance, meeting the right people, and having the ability to accept and move on with depression are your best and greatest gifts to help you through your emotional journey in life. As you read my story and it's just my story I cite no doctors or psychologists in my writings. I have personally found my own ways to deal with the emotional rollercoaster that my life has been. I am sure it will continue to be.

Another reason why, this time, instead of giving in and sinking into a massive depressive state, I have chosen to fight like I have never fought before. I have decided for myself and my family that they need me to still be here. My grandson needs his Nana. He is my inspiration, now and always. As I say to him each and every day: *"I love you to the moon and back, and all the stars in the world."* When I see his face and reaction every time, it gives me strength and most importantly, my reason to fight.

As Jelly Roll said: *"I believe in who we were is not who we are now. I believe that we can change. Who we are at any moment. I believe that people change. I believe that things can change."* Belief in yourself is always going to be your strongest asset.

If we could erase all our bad mistakes of the past, we would also erase the wisdom we have learned in the present. Remember the lessons you learn along the way. Don't remember the disappointment. I have watched many people over the decades treat me like I was optional. They showed me that I didn't matter. Believe me that shit changed me. I stopped loving people the way I used to. I certainly knew not to trust people so easily.

I never offer any explanation to anyone anymore. I realized that if they lost me, then so be it. Just know if you didn't stand up and fight for me when I needed you the most, I was no longer there to be taken advantage of. After a while, I realized that people liked me when I was quiet. I stopped questioning things. I just kept saying yes but that broke me more.

As I was walking through some parts of my journey, I came to realize that people loved the old version of me the one that was tired, confused, and so many times afraid to walk away. Now I hold myself differently. I speak differently. I have found my strength. I think twice before I say yes. I stopped showing up for the people who never checked on me or loved me for me. At some point, you need to stop explaining yourself to those people who never listened in the first place.

I had to stop believing I was the bad one in my life. I started healing, but then I also became the "wicked person" in everyone's life that I let go. Trust in your gut. Our brains always get fooled. Our hearts give in. But your gut will know when someone is lying. Behind each of us is a strong person. Each story will be different, but it is your story that changes.

You will fight battles no one will ever see. The weight we carry the weight of the world sits on our shoulders. Stop showing up for the ones who don't respect you, for the ones who have no sense of loyalty to you. Stop questioning your worth. The time is now to stop the betrayal by the ones you trusted the most. Silence will come when you realize the ones you thought loved you are now gone.

Your lesson learned is that sometimes the only person who's going to have your back is you. We all end up with fake friends that come and go out of our lives. Your own peace is what you will always be fighting for. You can never give what you don't have. Give your love to yourself that is worth fighting for. That becomes your power, as you have already lived through your own personal hell.

I was just a few years older than my grandson when I entered into a new dimension of what I thought reality was. My life was suddenly being altered in the worst way a child can go through. Sexual abuse is, and always will be in my mind, the worst experience a child of any age can go through.

In my day growing up, there was nothing around in regards to helplines, going to your parents, or just being able to talk to someone. Today, most kids are luckier. Today's society speaks loud about the issue. I am glad to see the change, at least in my days of living. Although still, in today's society, there is abuse of children that continues to happen. That is a hard thing to understand but it will always be a fight to end child abuse.

Through the following pages, I will walk you through the challenges I personally faced. I will walk you through how I dealt with them, or how long it took me to see a new insight into traumatic events. I will explain the emotional pain and the changes from who I was to who I have become. I will show you there is always a way to kick depression's ass.

This is not an easy journey to read about. It may bring a tear or two to your eyes. I share my story of personal hardship, my struggles, and my most personal inner emotions. Although my innocence was taken at a very young age as well as my older sister's that story I will come back to once my memory allows me to reopen the first traumatic event in my life.

It's so true with the saying, *"With time and age we lose our memories."* More importantly, the mind has a way of shutting down when a traumatic event happens. Sometimes we are lucky and forget about it for the time being, or by some grace of God we are able to close it into a memory and no longer remember. Almost like we wipe it out. Unfortunately, that event has a way of coming back. Through my journey, each one came back in full force to memory. Now, I have a hard time keeping good thoughts in and bad memories out. That seems to be the life of my depression.

As I begin my over-eventful life with you, please remember this is just my life and how I have personally dealt with my journey. My family had moved from a very isolated town into a bigger one, as my older sister needed to go to high school and our small town only accommodated up to grade 8. So off our family went once again for another move. Talk about walking into a strange world when you're not used to more than three streets or more than a few hundred people.

As I was still in grade school and raised Catholic, my brother and I were put in Catholic school. Up until now, I had been in split classes.

It's a chilly September morning and school is starting, so off we go. I walked into class late, as our parents were registering us that morning. The class suddenly went so quiet you could hear a pin drop on the carpet. The teacher, stern and "educated," looked at me and simply said, *"I believe you are in the wrong class grade 7, down the hall."*

I replied, *"I am in grade 6, and my brother is down the hall in grade 7."*

A look of astonishment came over her face as I stood there in the required dress code, but underneath I was still wearing my jeans. I was refusing to take them off. I hated dresses, and I hated even more that the way it was designed was not for girls with a chest.

I took my seat in class, and from the very first moment I sat at my desk, the boys stared so hard at me that the teacher had to move them to the front. That was the beginning of a horrible journey through grade school. Every day became a challenge. Boys always stared at my chest, made comments, and laughed at me. This would haunt me daily until I turned 21. I was bullied so badly that after grade 7 I wore sweaters and huge shirts. I refused to let anyone see my chest size. I was horrified growing up, my chest size didn't match the rest of me. I stayed at 100 pounds until I turned 47, except during pregnancies.

One day, getting on the school bus, I suddenly felt hands coming around me from behind. As I looked down, they were covering my breasts and holding on as tight as they could. I turned around with great force and kicked the boy between the legs. Suddenly, a teacher was yelling at me and another was grabbing my arm tightly. I was dragged into the office and asked to hold out my hands while the teacher struck them with a ruler. I was devastated and cried. I was so distraught that I even walked home.

By the time I got there, my parents had already been informed. Thinking they would at least ask me what had happened, I was crushed when they instead took the word of someone who hadn't seen what led me to kick the boy. The next day, I returned to school embarrassed and hurt that this was what Catholic school had turned out to be. I couldn't believe it.

The abuse from that boy continued through the entire year, with no resolution to stop his groping of my body. As time went on, more boys would join in on what they thought was "fun." It was a hard experience to endure, filled with daily ridicule over my breast size and my small frame. No matter how much I complained to my parents about what was happening, neither of them was in a place to know how to handle the extra pressure.

Another year passed, summer ended, and it was time to think about going back to the dreaded Catholic school once again. The fear that was already running through my mind had me on the brink of not being able to handle things at all. For the first time in my life, I felt a sudden fear unlike anything before. Emotionally and physically, I was petrified. My fear was so overwhelming, it completely took control of me.

No one would listen to me not about my emotions, not about my genuine concerns of not wanting to return to that school. Slowly, I began to cut myself across my wrist, over and over again. I managed to keep it up on a constant basis until one day, I left my bedroom door open and the babysitter saw me.

I started crying hard, begging him not to tell anyone. I begged him not to tell my parents. He said that as long as I stopped cutting, he wouldn't say a word but if I did it again, all bets were off. I still wonder, even now, why he didn't ask me why I was doing it. Why he didn't ask me why I was in so much pain.

I stopped cutting, but instead I began pushing all that emotional torment down into the pit of my stomach.

For the better part of my young life, I had been pushing all my emotions deep down. I tried, over and over again, to push my thoughts and feelings away. I learned how to fake my mood at a very young age. I learned far too early in life how to hide how I felt. I learned the hard way to keep my emotions in check. Best to keep how I felt to myself. It seemed to me, even then, that no one really cared about what I was going through.

As each day passed and things never seemed to get better, my parents were always fighting, and my mom was always extremely high on prescription drugs. Back to school I went, and the year was progressing like any other. The feeling of being lost and uncomfortable was still overwhelming. At least from time to time in grade 6 and 7 we each had a child we adopted in school. When you entered grade 6, you were paired with a kindergartener, and you would carry through with them the following year in grade 7.

One spring morning, Jason the boy I had adopted in kindergarten came up to me and said, *"I have to go get my mom from the airport today. It's going to be me, my brother, and my dad. We're surprising her at the airport."*

I said that sounded like the best idea I had heard in some time. I was still in school when the boys left to go pick up their mom. As the last class was starting after the afternoon recess, the teachers suddenly looked as though they were trying hard not to cry in front of 100 students. They were visibly shaken.

As we looked around for teachers to gather the younger ones, there were still none in sight. Some of the students from grade 7 stepped up and brought the younger students back to their classes. When the teachers finally returned, they clutched their rosaries tightly.

As they entered the classrooms, they asked us to return to our seats and told us we would all be called to the gym for an explanation. All of them had been crying it was clear from their faces and red eyes.

As we walked down to the gym, we couldn't help but stare at the teachers, trying to understand what they were holding back. Suddenly, the gym fell silent in a split second. No one had to be told to be quiet.

The principal stood before the gymnasium full of children. She cleared her throat, wiped the tears from her eyes, and spoke these words:

"It is with great sadness and grief that I tell you, just after lunch on the highway to the airport, there was a dreadful freak accident. It is with much sadness that I must tell all of you that we lost two of our students today. They were hit by a logging truck en route to pick up their mom from her trip. Sam was in grade 1, and James was in kindergarten."

School was let out early that day. Parents who could be reached were called to pick up their children. Sam had been my brother's adoptee, and James was mine. Neither of us knew how to deal with this new emotion this heartbreaking experience we had never felt before. Neither of us had lost anyone in our lives up to this point.

Our mother came to get us that day, as my brother had to go to the orthodontist in the next town. That meant we both knew right away we would pass by the scene of the accident. As we got into the truck, we told our mom what had happened, as we were both extremely upset over losing our "little people"the ones we were supposed to protect.

As we drove around Dead Man's Curve, my brother looked at me. I was crying, and he said, *"Maybe you should keep your head down when we drive by. It might not be cleaned up yet."*

Several times, I tried to close my eyes as we drove, but it was hard. I kept seeing the boys talking to me that very morning. Suddenly, the horrific scene was right in front of us.

The destruction to the truck was unbelievable. Even at that young age, I didn't think trucks could come apart like that. Parts of it were scattered all over the gully to the left of the highway. I looked at my brother, my eyes full of distress, and said, *"They should be on this side of the road, not that side."* I realized then that their dad must have misjudged the corner and not seen the oncoming logging truck. The back bumper was sticking out of the front window, and the front bumper was lodged in the back of the truck.

As we came to the end of the accident, we saw a bus full of people crying by the side of the road. Among them was the mother the wife who had just returned home from her trip. She stood there being consoled by others. At that very moment, I felt such loss, such heartache, such emptiness. It was more than I could handle. This was my first real experience of loss. Seeing the aftermath, the raw destruction, sent cold shivers down my spine.

Over the next few months, emotions ran hard and strong over the deaths of those three family members. The school held a service for all the children, but for many of us it was an especially painful experience. When the pictures of Sam and James were placed on the tables, tears flowed fast and uncontrollably from the majority of students. It was a sombre day, to say the least.

That day, I also saw my mother stoned in public for the first time. I was stricken with guilt, sorrow, and loss. The accident changed me that day and so did the actions of my mother.

I learned what heartbreak was, what it meant to lose a loved one. I learned how scared I was of death, and from that moment an overwhelming fear entered me and stayed persistent each and every time I had to deal with death from then on. Unfortunately, I had to start facing the death of students and friends from that point forward in my life. I used to have this old idea that death only happened when we got older. Was I naïve to think something like that? Probably. But because I never said anything about my fear and pain when it came to death, it only got worse the more people and friends I knew who passed away.

High school was even more painful. What a joke it was to think it would be different just because I was back in public school. The pressures were worse the amount of kids contending with one another was in the hundreds. I had just entered a new twilight zone I was by no means ready for. And like the rest of us, I had no choice but to move forward, just as everyone else did. Why should it be different for me?

Well, that perception didn't last long. In grade 8, we lost 10 kids I went to school with. In one night, 5 students died in a fire in an abandoned house. For days afterward, we listened to other kids describe the horror of what they saw while they stood outside the house, unable to get in. All the windows were boarded up, and something had fallen in front of the only door. People listened helplessly as the screams grew inside, then faded as the fire spread. They stood there and cried uncontrollably as 5 lives ended kids who had only just begun their journey in life.

More losses followed throughout my high school years.

The more death there was, the more depressed I became. My emotions became overwhelming to the point where I was physically ill. I suffered from massive stomach pain like it was on fire and being stabbed over and over. I went to my parents, but my mom, being a nurse, brushed it off as me just wanting time off school. But that wasn't the case at all. The pain got worse and worse. Eventually I developed a fever and was constantly throwing up. After months of this, my parents finally brought me to the doctor.

Sitting there in the office, my mom and the doctor talked about me as if I wasn't even in the room. The doctor didn't take my temperature, didn't do any tests, didn't even touch my stomach. She just looked at me and said, in a very stern voice, *"Stop wasting my time and your mother's. There are sicker people who need my attention. This crying wolf won't work."*

When my mom brought me home, I went straight to my room and cried for days. But the more I cried, the worse the pain became.

My emotions and heartbreak became unbearable once again. And like before, I resorted to my old way of numbing the pain. Old habits die hard. I began cutting myself again. Only this time I was older, a little wiser. I didn't use a kitchen knife. I stole a razor blade from art class, slipped it into my pocket a week earlier. Maybe deep down, I already knew I was coming close to giving up. What was the point of all this heartache, sorrow, and sadness I couldn't control? I was tired of hurting. Even more, I was tired of bottling everything up inside.

I couldn't see a purpose to life anymore. I was getting sicker, no one was listening, and every time someone just told me to "stop faking it." I was already lost in my own world, a young person with no one listening and not a soul who cared. People would later say I acted like I had "middle child syndrome." By far, that was not my issue. Yes, I was the middle of five children, but with foster kids and billets living with us, it was never about being "the middle."

After years of fighting, my parents decided to end their marriage. On the morning of my 15th birthday, I was walking upstairs when my father, at his wits' end, looked at me and said in an upset voice, *"Your mother or me?"*

I replied, *"Mom doesn't hit me. I choose her."*

He said, *"You and your mom have until the weekend to remove yourselves and find a place."*

I can still remember the heartbroken look on his face, the sadness in his eyes. For the first time, I saw my dad's inner pain. He went to each of the kids and asked the same question. By the end of that week, my mom, little sister, and I had moved into a very small apartment after a life in a house. The dismantling of the family unit sent us into a downward spiral that lasted decades.

A year went by, and my mother decided she needed to try something new. She uprooted my sister and me and brought us to Calgary. Talk about culture shock. I had spent a decade in a small town, and now I was dropped right into the middle of a fast-paced city life. One might have hoped the change would be good but it only got worse, in every way.

Mom was never sober anymore always high on prescription drugs, never there when we needed her. Suddenly, I was sicker than I had ever been. Of course, she made me go to school, insisting it was "all in my head." I cried, I yelled, I told her, *"No, it is not in my head, and I am not faking!"* Then I left for school.

The first class was in the gym. Right in the middle of running back to the centre line during warm-ups, I collapsed.

An ambulance had to be called. Because of a massive accident on the highway, the nearest hospital was backed up. The paramedics were told to take me to the nearest clinic for assessment. They wheeled me in on a stretcher, but before they could even move me inside, the doctor stopped them. He said, *"This girl doesn't look good at all. Why is she here and not at the hospital?"*

When the paramedics explained about the highway accident, he began to assess me right there. After only a few questions, he said I needed to go to the hospital immediately. He suspected I was suffering from a bleeding ulcer.

I had internal bleeding, and I needed treatment now not later. He got on the phone instantly, calling ahead to the hospital. After years of being in massive pain, unable to do most things day after day, all it took was one doctor, less than ten minutes, to save my life.

I spent the next three days in the hospital. When my mother finally showed up, she didn't even say she was sorry for not believing me.

Luckily, they didn't have to operate. They managed to use other means to stop the bleeding, and since then I've been on medication. When they first said surgery might be required, I begged them for another solution. I cried and cried until a hospital worker came to see me and asked why surgery was so devastating to me.

I told them, *"Because my mom had that surgery, and I don't want to end up like her sick, dependent, and never able to come off addictive medication. I'm already living that life with her. I don't want it for myself."*

I was only 16, and already I had a strong desire not to be here anymore. Life was such a struggle in every aspect of a young woman's life. I would watch my friends with their families, then go home and cry, asking, *"Why did I get the shitty end of the stick? What did I do wrong when I was so young?"*

When I visited my aunties and uncles and saw them with their kids, I would go home furious, jealous, and heartbroken. Why wasn't my mom like her sisters and brothers? By now, I was stuck, bewildered, and completely lost.

Somewhere along the way, I finally said, "Enough is enough." I was tired of my mom always being out of it, never functional. I was tired of the constant phone calls about bounced cheques, of eviction notices always being posted on the front door. I was tired of the trail of pills leading from her room to the living room to the bathroom. This was my life as sad and messy as it was.

At 17, I went out on my own, thinking anything was better than what I was living. Oh yeah, it was hard as hell being 17 in a big city by myself. I found a job, got a roommate, and we rented a place. Maybe it wasn't the best idea at the time, but it was my only option.

My roommate was older and of drinking age. Because I was more developed than most, we would dress up, go down to Electric Avenue, and party. Back then it was easy to get into bars, and before long, weekends of partying turned into drinking every other day. Before I knew it, I was becoming an alcoholic fast.

One night we were downtown again, having a few drinks and dancing, when suddenly my friend yelled, *"Those bitches are running off with our purses!"*

Without thinking, I jumped over a short railing and landed on one of the girls. She swung at me and hit me over the head with my own purse. Fear surged through me, but I channeled it into anger and swung back. I went too far, and before I knew it, there was blood.

Suddenly, I felt my arms being pulled forcefully behind me. Yep my ass was being arrested. They brought me downtown and booked me for assault. As the police took notes, they got to my date of birth. The look on the officer's face was priceless when I told him I was only 17.

I was released with a promise to appear in court three days later.

For those three days, my stomach hurt so bad I wanted nothing more than to go to the hospital just to escape the trouble I was in. Meanwhile, my mom lectured me endlessly, like there was no tomorrow. Since I was still a minor, I had to stay with her until my court date.

When the day came, we walked into the courtroom. My heart was racing, my hands were shaking, and sweat poured out of me like a river. My mom made me sit and listen to all the cases before mine.

Finally, my name was called. The judge looked down at me from his seat high above and said, *"Young lady, what made you get into trouble? You don't look like most of the kids I see come through here. There is a great deal of evidence of the assault you were part of last week. Is there anything you have to say?"*

I swallowed as hard as I could, but not a word would come out of my mouth. I was speechless and didn't know what to say. My mom stood up and said, *"I am her mom, and she has been more than upset over the last few days. I do think she is very sorry for the damage she caused to the young lady."*

The judge looked over at me and asked, *"Do you have anything to say for yourself?"*

I apologized from the bottom of my heart, crying uncontrollably. The judge suddenly struck his gavel and said, *"What reason, if any, should I not put your ass in jail?"*

I went numb all at once. I looked up at him in disbelief and blurted out, *"I'm pregnant."*

My mom looked at me and began to cry. The judge looked back at me and asked, *"Are you sure? Or is this a false manipulation on your part?"*

I said, *"No, I'm not lying. I'm telling the truth."*

I hadn't yet had any pregnancy tests done. I had always practised safe sex, but an overwhelming sense had come over me I knew I was pregnant. That same day, my mom took me to a clinic for a pregnancy test, and sure enough, I was right.

Talk about a life-changing experience in one day. I was devastated, filled with fear and anxiety like I had never known before. I was in disbelief and didn't know what to do. At the time, I was living on my own, heading down a very destructive path. I was an alcoholic at 17, a high school dropout, now pregnant and ashamed.

I had to grow up instantly. I had to make a choice for the future of my child. I went back to my place, packed everything, and moved back in with my mom. I had spent most of my life saying, *"Once I move the fuck out, I'm never moving back in."*

My upbringing had not been an easy one. At 17, I had no real memories of a happy time in my life. I could not recall a single moment where my parents said they were proud of me not even for the smallest things. I never got a hug, never felt arms open to give me love. That stopped when I was very young, for reasons I may never fully understand.

I hated being home. It was a constant headache, never knowing what was going to happen each day. For most of my life, my mom was not sober. She was addicted to Tylenol 3s and any other painkiller she could get her hands on. I never brought friends over. It wasn't worth the embarrassment of explaining my mother's behaviour when she was stoned out of her mind.

Every other month we'd come home to an eviction notice taped to the front door for everyone in the complex to see. Every so often, the cops would show up, ask for my mom, and take her downtown. She was forever writing bad cheques far beyond her means. A few times, I was called in the middle of the night to go get her. Picking her up was worse than when she was high the withdrawals were unbearable. The puking, the half-coherent conversations between bouts of agony.

And damn, if you want to talk about being scared for your life my mom drove every day high out of her mind, barely paying attention to the road. We were in so many fender benders, I lost count. The fear of being in a car with her driving still sends shivers down my spine. I'm amazed we survived. Too bad the laws were so flexible then. There were times she drove the wrong way down one-way streets.

Everyone has a different path they follow through life. Until people walk in my shoes, suffer my pain, and see the horrific images

I've seen, they shouldn't cast their judgment. Otherwise, I couldn't care less what people think of me.

After a while, I stopped reaching out. As I moved through life, I realized it was always one-sided. I stopped wanting the apology. Instead, I started wanting people to feel what I felt when they broke me. I wanted the weight of their actions to sit with them in silence, just as I was left with all the pain they abandoned in me.

Some days, when I feel lonely and worthless, I almost wish the people who hurt me would, at least once in their lives, feel the complete loss of my pain. Maybe not a wish but a hope. A hope that one day they suffer, so they can finally understand what they did to me. How they destroyed me. Loved ones have been the most heartbreaking part of all.

Some days are harder than others. My biggest drawback the reason I get hurt so much is that I truly care about people. I always think about how I can help, forever putting others' feelings first, never wanting to upset anyone. Inside, I hide the pain. I put aside my feelings, knowing the end would still be the same. And in the end, all that caring left me with silence. Forgotten. No one ever noticed the weight I carried.

There have probably been a thousand days when I thought, *"What did I do wrong to deserve this life? I didn't deserve this."* It always seemed that every time I took one step forward, someone shoved me three steps back. Growing up, I thought I was cursed. No matter how hard I tried, I couldn't catch a break. I watched people stumble into good things without even trying, while there I was giving it my all just to keep standing, still wishing one day I would be enough.

But nothing lasts forever. It's time to stop pretending things will never change. If you believe enough, they will. Start stepping away not because you've lost yourself, but because you've spent too much time trying to matter to people who never saw your worth.

Stop being an option. Stop being someone's safety net.

Every time I gave and believe me, I spent years giving everything all I ever received in return were empty promises. Don't be as foolish as I once was, begging for love and asking for acceptance. One day, you'll stand up and say, *"I'm leaving with nothing but my self-respect and my dignity."*

And when you do walk away quietly, calmly, unapologetically… and send a middle finger up as you go.

Chapter 5:
What you personally choose to do!

What a broad statement that is there are so many ways a person might respond when life keeps handing them a constant stream of traumatic stress. As the years have gone by, I have thought of many ways to continue, and many times I've thought of just calling it quits ending this emotional rollercoaster I never seem to get off of. It has been my biggest challenge, and it will continue to be my challenge for the rest of my life, after so many years of turmoil and never seeing the light at the end of the tunnel.

I decided to believe that maybe I was the stronger one out of all my family and friends. If anyone could endure it, why not me? Oh boy, did it ever happen over and over again. My family mostly stood by, not knowing what to do, or in most cases not even knowing what to say to make it better. At times, I think it was harder for some of them to watch than it was for me to live through.

As the years flew by, and the battles of traumatic events never stopped, I often thought of the movie *A Series of Unfortunate Events*. Every now and then I'd laugh bitterly and think, *"They should make that about my life a never-ending series of unfortunate events."*

The years passed, and the events never seemed to end. Learning to handle the pain, suffering, and heartache was in itself a battle deciding each time whether to go on, or to let it win. We all have choices in life; we all possess the power of free will. That alone should hold us higher. But always in the back of my mind was this truth: if I took the easy way out, what would be left? Only the broken pieces for my family and loved ones to pick up after me. That isn't fair not to them, and not to me.

There is a purpose for all of us to be here. As hard as it may be, with as little light as you might see at times believe me, it gets brighter and better. Time will not erase wounds, but it can help heal them. The mind never forgets the trauma, but you have the ability to change the direction in which you face it and how you deal with it. And if you cannot do it on your own, ask for help. Asking for help is even harder than surviving the trauma itself but it is necessary. When you're overthinking, remember this quote: *"Worrying does not take away tomorrow's troubles, it only takes away today's peace."*

Our deepest dreams don't wait for perfect timing. My night terrors demanded courage, sacrifice, and determination they forced me to refuse to die, but instead to fight. The world has doubted me more times than I can count. My life has been challenging, but I know my dreams will only survive if I fight for them. I have stood tall, and I tell you now chase your dreams relentlessly. Show everyone that nothing will ever stop a heart that burns with purpose.

Remember this: if someone believes they can find someone better than you, absolutely let them go. Never hold on to people who cannot see your value. In fact, show them the door and wish them well. Never chase someone who doesn't truly love you. Love should not be that hard. One day, the right people will show up, and they'll choose you not just once, but every single day.

We all want to feel loved. We all want to feel like we matter. When I was broken and hurting, I became so sad. I used to do absolutely anything for anyone else. I never wanted another person to go through what I've endured. It's crazy what a good person with a kind heart and soul will do for others. All I ever wanted was the same kind of respect in return.

That's what hurt the most. I gave and gave, everything I had, even my heart but all I ever got back was a broken heart and tears streaming down my face. I ended up with more pain, more emotional stress, and more anxiety.

We all want someone to treat us the way we treat them. But this is the world we live in a sad one. Over my life I've come to realize that the purest form of love is often overlooked. If people would stop to consider how their actions make others feel, they would show us just how much they really value us.

As you guide yourself through your journey, you learn to choose calmness over chaos. Finding peace becomes your ultimate priority. Surround yourself with people who are good for your mental health, your body, and your soul. That's part of growing.

Finding the right friends is a challenge. The friends you need are the ones who listen without judgment, who never speak with prejudice, who understand without pretense, and who love you without conditions.

But if you choose to sit in the dark, crying and worrying about your problems, you'll never bring them out into the light. You'll never fight the trauma by staying silent. Or worse, you could end up like me as a child surrounded by family, friends, and doctors who told me it was all in my head, who dismissed me as "crying wolf." Those early years were the hardest of all. I was screaming for help, destructive to myself, and yet no one paid attention. No one noticed my emotional distress.

I can say, sitting here as I write my story, that I fully understand the turmoil one goes through when living with depression. It is even worse if you don't know you have it when you just feel left out, like you don't quite fit into the world around you. You are not the only one to feel this way, and you certainly won't be the last. But you can change the direction of your fate. You can choose to cover it up, hide it from those who love you, or live your life in silence until one day you can no longer bear the loneliness or the pain deep inside. The truth is, no one can help you fix what they don't know is broken. As the old saying goes, *you cannot fix what isn't broken.*

Nowadays, it is much easier to get help for depression in a number of ways. Yes, at some point, some of us will have to try several different options until we discover what works best. I went through years of being alone, being told to "get over it" and "get on with life." When you are struggling with depression, those are the absolute last words you want to hear. My thoughts were always the same: *"Walk one mile in my shoes. Take my life and then see if you can just get over it and move on."* No, it is not that easy not for us. It's hard even for people who don't suffer from depression, so why are we expected to simply "suck it up"?

How you handle things will depend not only on your emotional and physical strength, but also on the support you get from your loved ones and your doctors. The most important thing you can do for yourself is not give up. Keep striving forward. If one thing doesn't work, try another and then another. Sometimes you may find yourself kicking and screaming just to get someone to help you. If that's what it takes, then kick louder and harder. Don't ever settle for someone telling you to "just get over it." Don't ever settle for someone saying, "It's all in your head." Yes, depression is in your head, but those are issues that need addressing and proper attention not dismissal.

Depression is one of the worst diseases you can face. Why? Because there is no real cure. Life, with all its traumatic events, is bound to give people depression in one form or another. Nowadays, a very large portion of the population suffers from it. Some experience emotional depression, some PTSD with depression, and others like me have lived with it since childhood. Sadly, many kids today are also suffering. Childhood depression often stems from family distress or from bullying in school and bullying has become one of the biggest triggers of all.

Too often we hear about another child taking their own life because they believe there is no way out of the pain. Suicide becomes the escape when they cannot find the right person, the right help, or the right way through the chaos. I've seen it throughout my life close friends and acquaintances clinging to their last thread of hope, only to have it ripped away. As children and preteens, so many of them felt hopeless, like they had no one to talk to anymore.

Kids today seem to have a different perspective on suicide. Some believe that by documenting their pain, they can bring change. And while some do make a difference, others don't. A parent's worst nightmare is having to bury their child. No matter the circumstances, the grief is unbearable. When the cause is depression, it's even harder because the parent is left asking, *"What did I do wrong? Why me? Why my child?"*

Some might say those children were angels sent to spread awareness. Others blame the parents, asking why nothing was done before it was too late. But it is never that simple. Unless you've walked in their shoes, you don't know. I was one of those children who gave up asking for help, because no one believed anything was wrong. That's one of the cruelest setbacks of depression you don't *look* sick. You don't *look* like you need help. Depression is the silent killer of countless good people every year.

Living with depression is like fighting a personal war. It is a constant battle of emotional torment and imbalance. It is a silent enemy that tears apart your soul and your sense of self. At times, the pieces feel too shattered to ever fit back together. Too often, hope is lost, and with it, the will to live. The emotional and physical pain becomes exhausting, and when all feels lost, giving up seems like the only solution. For some, it wins. For others, the fight becomes even stronger.

Over the decades, I have walked many roads to recovery. Some brought me to the edge of giving up, while others pushed me to try harder to find new ways to cope with the pain, suffering, heartache, and torment I was carrying both emotionally and physically. As a child, I begged my parents to listen, to hear me when I said I wasn't healthy and that something was wrong. The sicker I got, the louder I cried out, but it didn't matter. My family didn't listen. They didn't want to hear.

As a child, I couldn't understand why no one would listen. I couldn't understand why I was always pushed aside, as though I didn't matter. That's how depression works it convinces you that you are invisible, that you are not worth saving.

I was always made to feel like the lost soul, the black sheep of the family. Whether that was the intention or not, it's simply how life turned out while I was growing up. When my family no longer listened, that's when I first started cutting myself. It was the first time I felt no pain from depression. When I was caught and not by my parents I made a promise to stop. But still, no one listened. It had reached the point where it felt like no one cared. That was hard.

It didn't matter how loud I screamed or how much I begged for someone to pay attention it never worked. That's when I began acting out. I deliberately got myself in trouble, hoping my parents would finally notice I was hurting. I figured out young that maybe my only purpose was to take the shit in the family, to endure the suffering so no one else had to. But really what good did that do for my life? For a while, I tried directing my frustration, pain, and suffering into my school writing.

I had an English teacher who, for some reason, saw my pain. I became her challenge that year. She pushed me and pushed me to write. She gave me extra work in class, more than any of my classmates. She hounded me for the next two years of my education, drilling me to keep writing, asking me what I was thinking. I believe she knew I was suffering from something, though back then, depression wasn't openly discussed especially not in children. When I left town in grade 9, that was the end of my writing. I put my stories and poems in a box, left them behind, and never looked back.

Every now and then, I thought about those stories and poems. But I never searched for them, never felt the urge to revisit what I had written so many years ago. Would those words have changed my life if I had held on to them? I wish they could have, but in reality, they wouldn't have. Then, just a few weeks ago, my eldest daughter came to me holding a blue binder. My heart raced. My breathing quickened so fast I thought I might faint. She wasn't saying a word, but I felt my anxiety skyrocket. And then I realized why: it was *my binder*. All the stories, all the pain I had written down when I was young.

How my daughter got it, I never asked. I just took the binder, went to my room, and put it in the closet. One day, I'll open it. One day, I'll read what I wrote so long ago. Maybe by the time this story ends, I'll even share one or two of those writings here.

Life will always bring challenges, but it will also bring moments of purpose, of meaning. Because I went untreated for so long, lost within the disease, it got the better of me for many years. I made poor choices with my life, my career, my education, and even my self-respect. Changing how I thought and taking my life back has been, and still is, the hardest job I do every single day. There's no magic cure. There's no single pill to make us happy. But you can find what works for you.

You can find inner peace through acceptance and passion, rather than sinking into failure and misery. You are the only one who can take back control of your life. You are the only one who can make the difference you want, need, desire, and most importantly deserve.

People around you, especially those closest to you, cannot help change your direction if they don't know you're struggling. If no one knows you're broken, they can't help you stand back up. Friends and family can be your biggest supporters, but only if they know what's happening. I kept it a secret most of my life. To most people, I just seemed angry, miserable, always in a bad mood. What they didn't see was that depression was winning those days. Back then, depression wasn't spoken of, wasn't recognized, and you certainly weren't going to be diagnosed with it as a child.

Thankfully, today, more people are speaking out. Depression is no longer swept under the carpet. But still, many take the easier road they let depression win. And depression is one of the worst silent killers. Those who suffer truly suffer, and nothing seems to change the way the mind and body feel. The worst part is not having control over your emotions or your traumatic experiences. That's something we can never fully control. But what we *can* control is how we fight back against our depression and PTSD.

Yes, I've had those same feelings tired of hurting, tired of waking up another day. But each morning you open your eyes, remind yourself: you are in control. You are stronger than this. You are more powerful than it. Remind yourself that you are loved, that you are needed. Ending it won't solve the problem it will only hand it to everyone who loves you.

There were so many days in my life where I didn't think I could face another one. But when the next day came, and it wasn't quite as hard as the last, it reminded me that life can get easier. Your destiny belongs to you. Everyone is here for a purpose. Stand up now and find yours. Maybe it's finally your time to understand, to share your story, to help someone else. Pass on what you've learned to another soul who needs a guiding hand. Look at them and say, *"You can do this. I've got you. I'll help you through it."*

Teaching someone is the best gift you can give to someone who truly needs it. I remember how hard it was for me to accept that I couldn't believe what I was being told. I refused to accept that my head and emotional state weren't right. But they weren't not even close. I was on an extreme emotional rollercoaster every single day.

Feeling like you're trapped on a personal rollercoaster is almost impossible to get off. I was a young mom of two, recently separated from an abusive husband who constantly stalked me everywhere I went. One day, I called him and said, *"I'm not well. Can you take the kids for me?"*

He left, but when he came back an hour later, he gently lifted my daughter out of the car, then suddenly grabbed my son and **threw him up the stairs.**

I was in shock. Two of my friends one being my neighbor and the other my childhood best friend came over soon after. I told them what had just happened and that I wasn't feeling right. My body and mind felt completely detached from me. I was overwhelmed by anxiety, stress, and failure all at once.

They sat me down in a chair and said, *"Just rest for a bit. We'll watch the kids."*

I sat there crying uncontrollably. I couldn't stop. I was wearing a big purple sweater with a hood. I pulled the hood tight around my head so no one could see my face. Then I tucked my legs up inside the sweater and pulled the cord tighter. Wrapped up, hidden inside that bulky sweater, I suddenly rolled off the chair onto the floor.

For the next hour, I rolled around the house, laughing and crying hysterically at the same time. I was completely lost in a manic state.

As I started to come back to reality, I stood up and walked toward the front door. I looked at it, turned around and I swear, I saw my ex standing right there. In a flash of rage, I clenched my fist and swung with all my strength.

But I didn't hit him. I hit the metal cupboard in the kitchen. The pain shot up my arm, into my shoulder, and through every bone in my hand. It was so intense that it shocked me back into reality, snapping me out of the manic episode.

I had asked my friends not to call anyone, no matter what. I was terrified of losing my children if anyone thought I was having a breakdown. They kept their promise, though neither of them would ever want to go through that experience again. And I sure as hell wouldn't either.

That moment was enough to make me admit, at least deep down, that I had depression. But for years afterward, I still refused to accept it. To admit it felt like admitting something was wrong with me with my head, my emotions, my entire self.

My breakdown wasn't something I'd wish on even my worst enemy. It shattered me. It changed my mindset, my confidence, and my stability. I started crying over everything. I lost control of my emotions. One day I'd feel okay, the next I'd feel lost, convinced no one was here to help me. I began to believe everyone was out to get me. My anger grew. I was becoming more and more lost in my mental state, and the choices I made weren't good not for me, and not for my children.

Being so mixed up wasn't good. I started drinking. I went back to the bars whenever I could find a sitter. That's where I met someone new. A few months later, I found out I was pregnant again.

It wasn't what I needed not at all. But I didn't believe in abortion. I tried to make it work with him, but it wasn't long before I realized he was nothing but a **prime asshole.** His verbal abuse only grew worse as the pregnancy went on.

I had moved my two kids and myself into a small two-bedroom trailer. In October, the pipes burst, leaving me with no running water in the kitchen. You'd think he would fix it, but no. Not only was the water gone, the stove broke too. He left it like that. I cooked out of a single electric saucepan for months.

Finally, at eight and a half months pregnant, I'd had enough. I packed up the van, determined to leave. As I was getting the kids ready, that asshole stormed outside, got into the van, turned it off, pulled out the keys, and threw them into the snowy woods.

My body shook with stress. I called a friend, and she came to get me and the kids. I left everything behind. As we were leaving, his dad pulled up and asked what had happened. I told him. He was furious with his son and understood completely why I was leaving.

A few months after the baby was born, the same dumbass came crawling back, begging me to take him back. He promised things would be different. And like a fool, I let him in.

But it didn't last.

I had finally lost the baby weight and was starting to feel proud of myself again. I got a babysitter, made a romantic dinner, and dressed up. Hours passed, but he never came. I sat there waiting, my dinner cold, my hope fading. Eventually, I cleaned everything up and was about to change out of my outfit when he finally walked in.

I asked, *"Why are you so late?"*

He sneered and snapped, *"None of your fuckin' business. You're not my mother."*

He stopped, looked me up and down, and added with venom:

"And you look so damn unattractive."

I had an overwhelming sense that something wasn't right again. My head didn't feel good, and I said out loud, *"Not this time. The asshole is gone."*

The next morning, I got up, gathered all of his belongings, and carried them outside. I dumped everything into a huge pile in my front yard. My neighbor had just brought back some gas in my jerry can I'd asked for it, though I never told him why I needed it. He assumed it was for the lawn.

He was sitting in his living room when he looked out and saw me standing there, pouring gasoline over the pile of furniture, clothes, and belongings. He instantly opened his window and yelled, *"No! Don't!"*

He called my boyfriend and told him, *"Your shit is about to go up in flames. She's losing it."*

As the fumes rose, I realized something if I lit that match, he would win. He would succeed in destroying me. He would win by taking my kids away.

Everything ran through my mind all at once. I was broken down again by a man but this time, I wasn't going to let him win. I walked back toward the door. That's when I heard the sound of screeching tires.

He jumped out of the passenger seat, a bat in his hand. My only thought was: *Oh, hell no.*

I pulled the matches out of my pocket and shouted:

"Pick up your shit, get it off my lawn, and get the fuck out of our lives or I'll set it all on fire!"

The following day, my landlord came over and said, *"We need to talk."* I invited him in. As he stepped inside, he looked around and asked, *"Where is everything?"*

I explained, *"I gave my stuff away when my ex moved in. When I ended things, I had nothing left."*

He nodded and said he had watched the whole thing go down yesterday. Then he added, *"I have an idea for you."*

He had just finished building a six-plex in the next town and asked if I'd be interested in moving there to take care of it. I jumped at the chance. Within weeks, I was moving. I felt good about it a fresh start, away from my ex's interference.

Before I moved, I'd been seeing the doctor regularly since giving birth to my daughter three months earlier. I was in constant pain in my lower body and bleeding all the time. Each time I went, the doctor brushed me off: *"You just had a baby. Give yourself time."*

I kept arguing, *"No, it's not that. It's worse."*

Finally, after many visits, I got a referral to an OB-GYN in the next town. My longtime friend came with me. They performed a biopsy of my cervical bone to check for abnormalities.

By the time we were halfway home, I was keeled over in pain, bleeding heavily, as if I'd just given birth again. I was terrified. My friend was petrified too. She didn't have a license but knew how to drive. Since I couldn't even sit upright, she drove us home. She stayed with me for two days as I lay sick, in agony, unable to even hold myself up with three children to care for.

On the third day, just before she was going to leave, the doctor's office called. *"You need to come in right away,"* they said.

We looked at each other in shock. They had told us it would take up to six weeks for results. Now they wanted me back in immediately.

I called my neighbor to watch the kids, and my friend and I got in my truck to drive back. Our minds raced the entire hour-long drive. My thoughts spun endlessly my kids, my future, my life.

When I walked into her office just three days later, my friend held my hand, bracing me for bad news. My palms were sweating so badly that droplets hit the floor.

The doctor looked at me, sighed heavily, and said, *"I'm sorry to tell you this, but your results came back sooner and faster than expected. You have cervical cancer. You have a couple of options: chemotherapy, or a full hysterectomy."*

I wanted to collapse. I was twenty-four years old, a single mom with three kids.

My choices were devastating. I could go through a long, drawn-out process of chemo, always sick, losing my hair, and losing myself while my kids watched me fade. Or I could choose surgery. Instantly, I said, *"I'd prefer a hysterectomy and be done. I can recover in two months with help from friends."*

But the doctor, the only OB-GYN in my district, looked me straight in the eye and, in a cold, stern voice, said: *"I won't do that surgery. I don't get paid for it if you're under thirty-five."*

My friend exploded. *"What the fuck? Are you kidding me? This woman has been in pain for months. Everyone brushed her off because she just had a baby, and now she's at stage three and you'll do nothing? You're fucked up!"*

She helped me to my feet and dragged me out of the office. I collapsed outside, falling to my knees, crying uncontrollably. I couldn't stand. I couldn't even drive.

We finally got back home. It was pretty late in the day. I tried to sleep, but I couldn't. Every time I closed my eyes, I kept seeing my funeral. My kids were alone they had no one. I had black circles under my eyes so deep they almost seemed shut from crying all night.

I put on my fake face and got my kids off to school. Sitting down with my second cup of coffee, I suddenly said to myself, *"Oh, hell no."*

I picked up the phone book yes, the actual phone book, long before the age of Google and started calling every doctor within an eight-hour drive. I called and called. No one wanted to help me. No one was willing to save me. I was so lost, so broken, beaten down to the core.

Still, something told me to try one more number. For the first time in my life, it felt like someone was truly listening to me. As I told my story, her voice began to change. I could hear her crying as I explained how I didn't want to die, but I also didn't want to give up on my life or my children. When I finished, she said softly, *"Can you please wait one minute?"*

It was the longest minute of my life.

She came back on the phone and said, *"Can you be here tomorrow?"*

I didn't hesitate. *"Yes. Absolutely."*

That's how I met Dr. Penner the best person I ever encountered in my life. He took me on as a patient and did everything for free, as any doctor should. After all, it should always be the patient's choice what medical treatment they want.

He saved me. The process was hard and emotional. Those memories aren't the kind you want to keep, but they made me stronger. They made me want to live. They gave me a new way of looking at life.

Looking at life differently isn't always easy. Wanting something new isn't always good either. As the old saying goes: *"The grass isn't always greener on the other side."*

I had a friend helping me around the house, and over time we built a friendship that turned romantic. He was a good man. He provided well and took care of things when needed. I was happy. One day he popped the question. After a few years, I said yes.

When you get married, you think, *"Maybe this time it'll be for life."* But this was already my second marriage, and I wasn't even thirty yet. Within the first week, I noticed a change in him his attitude toward me and my kids was different.

We lived out of town, at least twenty minutes away. I worked near a restaurant, and the roads were terrible, especially when it had been snowing hard. That night, the snow was piled up, and the highway hadn't even been plowed. By the time I finally walked in the door, exhausted, he started screaming at me.

"Tell me who you're sleeping with!"

I was stunned. I lost it. *"Who the fuck do you think you are?"* I shouted.

He shoved me against the wall, then forced his hand down my pants, roughly touched me, pulled his hand back out, smelled it, and sneered:

"You're lucky today."

I collapsed to the floor, shaking so badly I could barely breathe. My mind raced: *Who the hell did I marry?*

I pulled myself up, threw blankets at him, and yelled, *"Go fuck yourself!"* I didn't speak to him for days.

Sometimes people take longer than others to learn. That's me in a nutshell. Once again, I gave in to a promise his promise that it would never happen again.

I swore no man would ever hit me or touch me wrong after my first marriage. But only two days later, we were sitting at the table when he looked at me with a cold expression and said, *"I want something different. I want you to go to the bar tonight, pick someone up, and bring him home so I can watch from the closet."*

I was furious. *"One day you accuse me of cheating, and now you want me to actually go fuck someone in front of you? Are you insane?"*

I stormed into my room, shaking so hard I started to vomit. My mind raced in terrible ways. *What the hell did I do marrying him?* I felt so lost, completely out of control of my emotions. I couldn't stop crying. I felt like a failure.

I had only been married five months.

The next day, I woke up in a trance. It felt like my mind was floating outside my body.

For the next few weeks, the cycle never ended. One day he accused me of cheating. The next, he was calling me a slut, a whore, tearing me down until I felt beaten inside and out.

His best friend came over one day and found me crying in bed, looking sick. I hadn't eaten in days. I broke down and told him everything the accusations, the names, the emotional abuse. He punched the wall so hard his hand went through it. He turned to me and said, *"He asked me to partake… and I told him, 'How could you do that to your wife?'"*

A few more days went by. Then a couple of friends stopped by to say hi while they were in town. We sat having coffee while the kids played. My husband called and heard voices in the background. Immediately he accused me of fucking someone.

I snapped, *"Talk to them yourself."*

He did. But no sooner had I started another pot of coffee than he came storming through the door.

This man was supposed to be 55 kilometers away, working graveyards in another town. Instead, he had flown home just to catch me only to find us sitting with coffee and kids laughing in the background.

For hours, he yelled and raged while my friends left in utter disbelief. The children were woken up again and again by his screaming.

One day, he wanted me to go to the bar and bring home a stranger so he could hide in the closet and watch. The next, he was calling me a slut for being late.

I could never win. No matter how hard I tried, no matter how much I begged to be believed, my innocence didn't matter.

Not one single person ever really listened to me.

I got up the next morning humiliated. My heart was racing faster than I could breathe. I sent the kids to school on the bus and set up my youngest with something to play. This time, I owned everything house-wise. I had promised my children never to put them in that position again. My husband had come into this marriage with very little. There were a few things we had gathered over the years, but I decided he could have it all.

As he slept, I gathered his things, carried them out to the front lawn, and piled them up. Then I went into the room, threw a bucket of cold water on his sorry ass, and shouted, *"Get the fuck up! Get dressed and get the fuck out today!"*

He got dressed, and as he passed the window, he saw everything he owned soaking in the pouring rain. I had already called a few buddies over to help remove him, and they came, cleared him out, and changed the locks.

I was so broken by this point that I thought of myself as an even bigger failure than before. Damn my marriage hadn't even lasted six months. I was angry, too, furious at being treated this way. *Where the fuck was this man before I married him?* How dare he change the moment a piece of paper said we were bound?

To be honest, I had that gut feeling from the very beginning. Because of my first failed marriage, I had doubts. But I swallowed them, ignored them, pushed them aside. As I walked down the aisle well, more like that pathway and bridge I knew deep inside that something wasn't right. I should have listened. I should have trusted my instincts the first time.

The feeling of complete and utter failure, on top of already living with depression, was heavier than I could carry. It made my mind, body, and soul collapse completely.

It took time, but eventually I pulled myself up and brushed myself off. With time, I began to learn more about myself. I began to think, *I need to do something.* After all, I was now a twice-divorcée with three children to raise.

What do you do when your brain, emotions, and life are all messed up? Sometimes you don't even realize you're breaking down. Sometimes you don't realize your thoughts aren't right. *Should they be right?* Some would wonder. Damn, I wondered myself most days.

There is never an easy solution for anyone's problems. With depression, holy shit, it's worse. I say worse because I've been medicated for the last 15 years, and now I'm on the strongest side of it. I'm not willing to add more medication to my list. I once added Lorazepam in the smallest dose, and it fucked me up even more.

Already broken by my own thoughts, that extra little pill pushed me further over the edge. It screwed me emotionally, physically, and most of all mentally. If I wasn't already messed up, that drug turned me into someone I would never normally be.

And what did I lose? I lost everything that meant the most to me. I lost everything that brightened my day. I lost the happiest part of my life. I lost it all being scared, mentally shattered, and emotionally crushed.

Yeah, maybe you're wondering what I mean by that. The truth? The thought of suicide became my only thought. Constantly. I would look next door. I would listen for my grandson's little voice, stretching my ear as far as I could, just to remind myself he was there.

Maybe, over time, you stop talking to the people who hurt you the most. And that's okay. You can still wish them happiness from a distance. You've made it this far keep moving forward, even if it's only one small step at a time.

When you see yourself moving forward, make peace with what you've left behind. Let it go. Release it from your heart. As you walk down a new path, you may miss people, but you won't miss the pain they caused.

As you grow, your perspective changes. Even toward the ones closest to you. Start to pray for their healing, and at the same time, wish for your own dreams to come true. Thank them if you must for being part of your life. But remember this: you will never mean to them what they meant to you. At your best, you will still never be "good enough" for the wrong people in your life.

When you reach the absolute worst point in your life, one day you'll finally be right for the right people. One day someone will hold your hand, see your effort, and honor your growth. Someone will walk with you on your journey. Someone will light your way.

Pour your life into the friends who pour life and happiness back into you.

Over the years as a parent, I can't count how many times I had to hide my tears. I swallowed my pain, pulled every ounce of strength I had inside me, and kept moving.

As a mother, as a woman, the only thing we can do is try to keep the hearts of the ones we love whole. It was hard as a young mother already traumatized by hundreds of events but I always wanted my children. My children needed me. They needed a safe place, a shelter, a home.

Years later, I'm still dealing with drama from my own children. Sad, but true. And more importantly, if I could knock them both into next week for the mental, emotional, and physical abuse they put their own children through all because they were mad at me I would. Without hesitation.

I am more than disappointed. I am ashamed of their actions.

Believe that one day, someone will walk into your life and change everything. They will raise your standards, lift your spirit, and most importantly, they will make you laugh like you've never laughed before. Don't let it scare you. I did, a few times. And those times, I believe I lost a helping hand that could have changed my path. But when you meet this person, the fear of losing them will disappear.

When you're working through cleaning out the bad parts of your past, ask yourself: have you deleted all those photos that remind you of that trauma? I haven't. I don't look at them often, but I also haven't erased them. They're reminders of how I was hurt, reminders not to trust certain people again. They are only frozen memories of a time that nearly broke me. To relive them would mean to relive the trauma I worked so hard to overcome. So, I leave them. Untouched.

They remain quiet reminders of what was, maybe proof that a part of me still cares, or maybe proof that I haven't quite let go. But it's time. Time to let go and start becoming the person I want to be.

Sometimes the heaviest things you carry aren't in your hands they're in your heart. Pain is always the unspoken part of our battles, the part no one ever sees. A thousand times we've said, *"I'm okay,"* when deep down we're not. We push the feelings down just to make it through the day. On the surface we function, but inside the soul is exhausted.

Not exhausted from life itself, but from carrying the burden and pain alone. That's when you realize you don't actually need much. Just a little peace. A little quiet inside a loud, aching heart.

Remember this: when someone tells you about their past, it's not because they want your pity. It's so you can understand why they are the way they are. Just like you, they've been shaped by their journey. You may be broken some days, but you are never hopeless.

Some days, nothing hurts more than wiping your own tears, knowing you can't tell anyone the truth behind them. There are still weeks where I reach my lowest at least twice and that's when I distance myself from everyone. That's when I hurt most.

Something I've learned along my journey is that you need to find yourself and you need to let go of the people who constantly bring you down. Yes, even if they are family. You can't choose your family, but you can choose better people to become your family. People who won't hurt you. I'm still searching, but I'll never give up on wanting better for myself. I deserve better than what I've gotten from my family. That's for damn sure.

My biggest regret in life is my marriage. I was searching for love mostly because I never felt loved as a child. Damn, my first marriage turned abusive fast. After a mental breakdown, I finally walked away with firm help from others.

You see, I was never late for anything. Then one day, I was. My best friend walked to my house to check on me. She found me huddled in a corner, my kids beside me.

I was suffering from sleepless nights, fighting battles no one could see, begging for help. My neighbors lived close close enough to hear my cries but no one extended a hand, no one called the police. Instead, I endured a night of pure hell. Abused mentally, abused physically, while my two little ones watched. They woke in the middle of him punching holes down the hallway walls.

For years after, I was consumed with endless frustration, heartache, and mental suffering. Splitting up wasn't easy. I used to be one of those people who would say, *"Just walk away. Just leave."* But when it's you in that situation, full of fear, watching your family break apart nothing is simple. And by the end, I didn't even want to fix it. That relationship crumbled into nothing.

But I left. I stood back up on my own two feet. I moved forward.

It was hard, raising three kids alone, cleaning, cooking, working trying to do it all. And then came another blow: stage 3 cervical cancer.

I was already stressed about moving towns, raising two children and now a newborn. After fighting for the treatment I needed, after endless traumatic appointments, after begging someone to help me no one should ever have to go through what I went through.

I believed I survived only because I had to raise them.

Even though it's been more than 25 years since cancer, that journey still broke me. It broke me emotionally, physically, and spiritually. It took over a year for me to climb out of the depression. Over a year before I smiled again.

But one day, my son came up to me and asked, *"Is the old you coming back? I miss her."*

My heart shattered. My soul shattered.

Not only was I fighting depression and cancer, I can almost say for certain I also had postpartum depression piled onto my already traumatic life. My world was in complete turmoil.

Pulling myself together every day was exhausting. Every morning felt like a losing battle before I even opened my eyes.

But somehow, I got back on my feet. One day at a time. And then, I found myself doing something ordinary again catching up on weeks of laundry.

Not only was I tired, but I was hungover for the first time in years. A friend came to spend the day with me it was finally a day of peace. But as I got home from doing laundry, I started to hear this god-awful screaming. My neighbor came running through my open door, tears falling onto my floor. She couldn't breathe. She couldn't talk. I sat her down until she finally managed to tell me she couldn't get the bathroom door open and couldn't find her man.

My head was pounding so hard, my anxiety was through the roof. It had only been two weeks since we all moved in I hadn't even had a chance to meet the neighbors. I pushed with everything I had, but the door wouldn't budge. I called the police and the ambulance, but my focus was on getting that door open. Finally, I managed to break in. He was so cold almost purple. His hand was stiff.

Watching and waiting for a body to be removed is a long, grueling process. It takes hours of people coming and going, people outside taking pictures. Finally, after five hours, I had to ask them to remove the body before all the kids got home. It was heartbreaking to watch the entire process, to see someone you just met sitting on your couch, completely losing it and there's no way to help but to sit beside them and offer what little comfort you can.

Sometimes your patience and love for another person come into focus, especially when you're trying to soften the hurt you're about to cause. Not by your fault, but by an accident. Believe me dealing with that kind of pain, the truest loss, is the hardest emotion to come back from.

I have come across death in many different ways. Each time, it has never been easy. It will never be easy. Death becomes the hardest truth there is absolutely no coming back. The biggest wish in the world cannot change the outcome of loss. The pain is real, and the impact is overwhelming. Death is never easy, not even for the cold-hearted.

For years, I was hesitant to be with anyone. I carried a fear I couldn't even put into words. Trusting someone wasn't part of my vocabulary anymore. As the years pressed on, I began to open up a little at a time. Then one day, when my friends and I went to the bar, we met some really nice guys.

Skip two years, and I finally agreed to marry again. I always thought in my head that I needed to be strong for my kids that I needed to give them a good role model to look up to. Once I said "I do," well…I had never been so blindsided in my life. I had been through some extremely harsh things, but this was beyond unfathomable.

I truly thought I needed a new life with this man, someone I had known for three years. Not once in those three years had I seen the person he truly was. One day, I came home about fifteen minutes later than usual. I walked into the house, and all of a sudden, he was yelling and screaming at me, calling me every name in the book. I was stunned. Furious. Like, *what the fuck?*

A few days later, he asked me if I would go to the bar that night. I said no and asked why. He literally said, "I want you to go pick up a guy, bring him home, and fuck him while I watch."

I know. *WTF, right?*

The cocksucker kept asking me to do this constantly. He would pressure me to sleep with someone, then the very next day, call me a slut and accuse me of cheating.

Several months went by. My wellbeing and mental health were completely drained. Did I ever go to the bar and pick someone up? Not even when I was single. But the pressure, the abuse, the mental torture I did end up in threesomes a few times. No, I didn't have a choice. Sometimes, it felt like the only way to get him to stop.

Finally, I broke down. And no, it wasn't the kind of breakdown that brings healing it was the complete collapse of my soul.

This was my second marriage and I wasn't even thirty yet. How sad is that? How embarrassing, looking into my children's eyes and seeing their disappointment. Another broken family. More broken promises from me that things would be different this time.

The sense of loss, the sense of failure it's one of the hardest things to recover from. Those feelings are brutal when you have children involved. No matter how hard you try to shield them, they still get hurt.

When you see true disappointment in your children's eyes, you see their sense of loss too. They had gotten emotionally attached. They even had a stepsister. And then it was all gone.

Growing up, all I wanted was a happy family. I didn't want to give my kids the broken home I came from. At least my parents only did it once. Me? Well, shit a few more heartbreaks for us all.

Chapter 6:
Getting Back Up Is Your Only Choice!

If there is one thing I have learned through this inner journey, it's that each time I had an emotional upset or a complete, utter breakdown, it did get easier over time to pick myself back up. There were certainly my share of upsets and breakdowns where I wanted to give up. I wanted nothing more than for the pain and suffering to go away.

Then one day, I woke up with a belief maybe, just maybe I suffer to bring awareness, to bring strength to those who don't have as much, or any at all. I started to believe that if I suffered, then none of my family or friends had to. I thought that if I could keep the pain to myself and keep my siblings free from it, I could be happy or at least happier.

Don't get me wrong, I've had my share of breakdowns and traumatic events well enough for several people and I am still here. A week ago, I didn't think this way. I thought much differently. I was willing to give up, to let my weaknesses take over, and I lost control for a few days. I cried and cried. Then I heard my teacher's voice, like I was back in 1985, and here I am. I have fallen many times over the last thirty years, but each time I have found the strength to stand back up and decide to fight again.

One of my first manic episodes happened when I was a young mother of two, finally splitting up from an abusive marriage. I had tried several times to leave my husband, but it isn't as easy as people think not when children are involved, not when you already feel like a failure because you couldn't keep the family unit together. I finally decided to end the marriage by committing adultery with one of my friends. That was finally enough for my husband to leave me alone.

Even then, though, he stalked me every chance he got. I took him to court and got a restraining order, but that didn't help. It only made things worse.

One day, he had visitation, and my two girlfriends were over. Suddenly, my body didn't feel right. I didn't feel right. Something was wrong with me my whole body was off. I was scared, becoming an emotional mess fast. I called him to ask if he could keep the kids just a little longer. *No way,* he said and within ten minutes, he was at my house. He swung my son out of the car by the arm. I lost it, yelling at him, but I quickly took the kids inside while my friends got him to leave. A few moments later, I turned to them and said, "I don't feel good."

I sat in my chair to think, and before I knew it, I was curling myself into a ball. I was wearing a big BOCA sweater, two sizes too big. I pulled the hood tight so you couldn't see my face. I pulled my legs up inside, tied it even tighter, and started rolling around my living room in a ball.

I did this for hours while my friends tended to my children. I made them promise not to call an ambulance I didn't want to lose my kids because of a breakdown. They kept their promise and let me have my emotional collapse. Hours later, I finally pulled myself together, got up, and cried like I had never cried before. Emotionally, I was drained. My thoughts and feelings felt detached from who I was, like I was split in two.

The next few years only brought more hardship, more emotional torment than I could handle most days. For a very long time, I didn't smile no matter what I did, no matter how hard I tried. I couldn't change the inner feelings I had succumbed to.

It was a constant struggle to get out of the emotional rollercoaster my life seemed to be. I struggled daily just to get up and put one foot in front of the other. I was already a single mom of two kids when I found myself pregnant again. Was the relationship I was in normal? Hell no. I was emotionally fucked up, and for a moment of weakness, I needed human touch something to remind me I was still human, still a woman.

I tried continuously to make it work for the sake of the unborn child. But it was an extremely hard pregnancy. The man I was with was an arrogant asshole. I had finally lost some weight, and one night, I wanted to feel romantic. I dressed in a black teddy with a short silk robe. He looked at me and said, *"I find you so sexually unappealing."*

I was horrified. The very next day, I packed everything he owned in the house and dumped it in the front yard. I called him at work and said, "You have one hour to get here or I'm going to light your shit on fire."

That day, I decided to take my life back. I stood strong. Maybe it wasn't right to threaten to burn his stuff, but for once, I stood up for myself. I said, *"I will not take this anymore."*

That was the last day I felt sorry for myself in that relationship. Whether I felt like a failure or not, I was done.

I gave notice on my place and moved to the next town. I needed a new start for my children and for my own emotional well-being. As hard as it was, I had to do it for them, and for me. I felt trapped in that town. Twenty years there had given me nothing but depression. The constant gray, depressing weather only made things worse.

I moved only 55 km away, but it felt like there were hundreds of miles between me and my old, sad life. I had only been there a few weeks when I started to feel different. My body was hurting in a serious way. I went to the doctor, and she decided I needed to be seen by a specialist. I had a biopsy done.

I was told prior to the procedure that it might cause some bleeding once I started moving around. Within twenty minutes of being home, I was bleeding heavily cramping worse than I had ever experienced before. It was worse than labor. The pain was unbearable. The only thing I could do was curl into the fetal position.

By the next day, the bleeding had eased slightly, but the pain intensified. I could hardly move. I couldn't take care of my children. For the next few days, I took it easy, following the doctor's orders. She had told me it would take a few weeks to get my results.

But within the first week, the doctor called and told me to come in as soon as possible. Terrified, I went with my best friend. I was scared shitless. Sitting in the waiting room, my hands were sweating, my legs bouncing up and down like a drumbeat.

The doctor walked in, sat at her desk, and opened my file. Clearing her throat, she looked at me and said, "I'm sorry to inform you, but you are at Stage 3 cervical cancer."

My heart sank deeper than it ever had before. I was in shock. I had three little kids. I was a single mom. My mind was racing so fast I could hardly catch up with what I had just heard. My body went weak, and I thought I might pass out until I suddenly felt a hand holding mine tightly. My friend hadn't let go.

The doctor gave me a few minutes to regroup. When I finally found my voice, I looked at her and asked, "What are my options?"

With a blank look, she said, "Two options." She went through her speech and then finished with, "I will not do your surgery because I don't get paid. You will have to find another gynecologist to perform the surgery, if that's what you want. Or you can go through chemotherapy. That option is there."

"What? Fuck no!" I thought.

My head was spinning. Slowing it down wasn't an option. *Stage 3?* For months, I had been complaining about the pain only to be brushed off by doctors telling me I "just had a baby" and my body needed time to heal. That got me nowhere. And now this? Getting results four weeks earlier than expected, only to be told the doctor wouldn't operate because she wouldn't get paid? I was furious.

The next few days, I cried myself to sleep. All I could think of were my poor kids. I was too young to die. I had just started to get into the routine of being a single mom, and now my life was turned upside down in a matter of minutes. I had to fix this for me, and for them.

After days of calling around to towns everywhere, I finally got a sympathetic nurse to listen. She put her doctor on the phone. By the grace of God, that day, someone actually cared someone willing to save my life and give my children a chance to still have their mother around.

Believe me when I say it was hard to get over this experience. To be told I was "too young." To have months of doctors ignoring me. To hear people who swore an oath to help say no because of my age. It took me over a year to stop being so angry, and even then, it was difficult.

Hardest of all was explaining to my children that I was very sick. My son, especially he had begged me for a baby brother. For two months after I had my youngest, he wouldn't go near her, wouldn't kiss her, wouldn't even look at her. He was angry. He wanted a brother, and he felt betrayed by me. I had promised him, "Maybe one day, when things are better." Had someone listened to me sooner, maybe things *would* have been different.

Finally, spring came a new year. I wanted to bring better memories for my kids. A friend of mine asked me to join his softball team; they needed a girl and a pitcher. If there was one thing I was always good at, it was pitching. My dad had taught me when I was young, and he taught me well. Over the years, I had perfected my technique.

The season was going great we entered tournaments, played weekly games, and had fun.

Until one day.

We played against a team that wasn't there for fun. They were hard, rude, and aggressive. A friend of mine had come to watch that day. The other team started giving me a hard time not just for being a female pitcher, but because I was striking out every asshole who mouthed off at me.

By the top of the 6th inning, their coach shouted to the batter, "Hit the bitch!"

My catcher immediately ran up to the mound, called the infield in, and said, "We need to change pitchers they're going for your head."

To put it in perspective: I stood five feet tall, weighed maybe a hundred pounds. The hitter? Over six feet, at least 240 pounds, with a metal leg brace and a pitch runner.

My attitude in that moment was: *no way*. Who the hell would deliberately target a pitcher female or male? And shit, I was so small. I refused to play in fear. Instantly, my anger boiled: *how fucking dare you!*

I shouted to my team: "Everyone, get into your places. Let's play some fun ball!"

I said it so loud, I'm sure the next field over heard every word.

I took my stance, inhaled deeply, and let go of the pitch. I knew if I threw more inside, I'd have less chance of being hit in the upper body. I followed what I was taught. But as soon as the ball left my hand, I tried to brace myself there wasn't enough time.

The batter hit a direct line drive. It smashed into the left side of my kneecap. The impact lifted me off the mound and threw me behind second base.

My shoes were still on the mound, but I was not.

I screamed in agony. I couldn't feel my left leg. Instantly, my teammates rushed to me. One tried to straighten my twisted legs my swollen left leg had crossed awkwardly behind my right. Another tugged at my track pants, desperate to see the damage. I screamed louder as they tried.

Then, all hell broke loose.

The entire field turned into a battlefield. Men from my team went after the batter and the coach who told him to aim for me. Fists flew everywhere. Pretty much everyone, from players to spectators, got dragged into the chaos. Blood covered the dirt. Even players from the other field ran over to help break it up, horrified by what they were seeing. Women in the crowd ran to me, crying hysterically at the sight of my knee.

Instead of just one ambulance, it felt like every police car in the town showed up.

I was rushed to the hospital. Surgery was immediate. The damage was bad. And that was only the beginning I endured four more surgeries after that hit. For ten years, I lived with unbearable pain and constant swelling, fighting and fighting to get a knee replacement.

I finally won my case. I was finally approved for surgery. After years of suffering unable to work, unable to ride bikes with my kids, unable to live normally I had hope again.

The process was long: psychological testing, pre-surgical assessments, paperwork, recovery plans. But it was happening. For the first time in years, I felt relief.

Two weeks before surgery, I went in for my last check-up. My childhood friend, the same one who'd been with me when I got my cancer diagnosis, came with me. We sat nervously in the office.

Then the doctor walked in.

I didn't recognize him. He wasn't the one who'd been scheduled.

I stood up. "Uh, no. Where is the other orthopedic?"

They told me his work visa had expired he had gone back to Africa. "I'm the one taking over his caseload," the new doctor said.

I sat down, my whole body sinking with dread. My friend saw the devastation on my face.

The doctor opened my file, asked a few questions, then, in a cold, detached tone, said: "I will not do this surgery. I will scrape your knee clean. You have no meniscus. You'll always be bone on bone. Or I could take part of your hip and use it to give you cushion."

My body shook. My chest tightened. The rage and hopelessness hit me like a tidal wave. This was happening again. Just like with the cancer.

I cried hysterically. "How can you do this to me? I did everything I was told. It was arranged! You can't "

But he didn't care. His decision was final.

I was told to leave his office. To "find another doctor."

I collapsed into days of sobbing. Depression swallowed me whole.

For years, I walked around in a daze, my knee swelling to twice its size every day. Work was impossible. Life was impossible. The pain consumed me. And just to add to it, I had a boyfriend at the time who blamed me for everything the lack of sex, the lack of housework pushing me aside for his own needs, ignoring mine.

Then, out of nowhere, someone came back into my life.

My ex-husband's best friend. The best man at my second wedding.

We had kept in touch over the years, talking whenever we crossed paths. He was always kind. Always steady. One day, during one of our conversations, he looked at me and said quietly:

"I have to be honest with you. I think I've fallen in love with you."

I was shocked. Flattered. And for the first time in my life speechless.

These were happy days for a while. But then my man was in a work accident that mangled his lower leg. That accident didn't just break his body it broke us. It was the beginning of the end of our twelve-year relationship.

His pain became our nightmare. We both suffered, and it consumed us. I went from battling depression to also living with PTSD, and so did he. I buried myself in everything outside the home just so I wouldn't have to be there. And when I was home, I hid in my room. I started becoming the kind of mom I swore I'd never be. My emotional and physical health crashed hard, and I couldn't stop it.

Those days of being a bad mom are some of my biggest regrets. I can never change them just like I could never change my own upbringing. I was trapped in my emotions, my thoughts, my fears. I lost sight of the person I was meant to become. I failed myself, and I failed my kids. I had promised I wouldn't be like my parents, but somehow I became worse. Detached. Untethered from who I truly was. I tried to keep up appearances, but inside I was broken. I cried, I lashed out, I made choices out of fear instead of strength.

That time also cost me my relationship with my mother. My father and I had never been close for many reasons, but when he finally retired, he deserved peace. Instead, my mother dragged him back into court. I thought it was unfair she had chosen her addictions, chosen her life, chosen not to quit the pills. Why should he still be punished twenty years after their split?

I stood up for my father. I wrote him a statement of support.

My mother instantly disowned me.

She stripped me of everything, including her role as a grandmother. She never came back to my home again. Ten years later, when I went to help my grandma, I saw my mother again still clawing, still bitter, still trying to manipulate.

Betrayal has been a constant in my life. Over and over, from people who should have been my safe place. It doesn't just take your mental strength it robs your trust, your innocence, your belief in love and loyalty. Those wounds leave scars you can't ever fully erase. They show up in night terrors, in sudden flashbacks, in a silence that suffocates you.

The pain of being hurt by the very people who said they loved me will never stop haunting me. They hurt me young, and they kept hurting me for years.

I used to sit quietly, wiping away tears, asking myself what I did wrong. Why did I deserve this? My family gave me their coldest moments, and I tried every day to earn warmth that never came.

But here's what I've learned: family doesn't have to be blood. If "family" is the cause of your pain, your silence, and your fear, then family isn't family at all.

I have fought to survive. I've thrown punches life never saw coming. I wasn't given anything at birth I had to fight for every ounce of my life. The fears that stay the longest are the broken heart, the exhausted spirit, and the lost soul. And let me tell you there's a whole quiet club of us who know exactly what that feels like.

Now, I choose to rise like a phoenix. I won't break under the pressure anymore. I'll show them how wrong they've been.

Some people think depression just means staying in bed all day. And yes, sometimes it does. But other days it looks like dragging yourself up to brush your teeth while your eyes are still swollen from crying the night before. It looks like trying to talk while your voice cracks because it's barely holding on. It looks like standing there silently begging for someone anyone to reach out a hand.

I once came across a piece from *My Heal Time* called **Hard Truths**, and it summed things up perfectly:

Some things you will never fully heal from. And that is not a failure. Not because you are broken. Not because you are doing something wrong. But because some pain stays. Some stories are meant to leave a mark. Expecting to erase them is not healing that's denial. Healing isn't about forgetting. It's about building a life that still feels meaningful, even when you're carrying what hurt you.

Chapter 7:
Finding Inner Peace with Depression

Talk about a bold statement for a chapter but for what it's worth, and for the challenges we face with depression, it about sums it up. This will be your hardest and most challenging battle to ever control in your life. I fought and I battled for years, day in and day out, month after month, year after year. You become numb to the hurt, to the pain, to the discomfort from depression, until most days you simply stop caring.

Some things I've learned along the way are this: I would rather be hated for who I truly am than be loved or adored for someone I am definitely not.

Learn to live by the saying *what you see is what you get.* You no longer have to change to suit people's expectations of who they want you to be. You must learn to change for yourself. You need to stop putting your trust in people who don't give you the same respect and loyalty.

As you move forward, remember this:

The moment we go quiet, suddenly people care. Nah they're only missing the light that used to shine when you were around. They never truly see the storms we walk through daily, carrying heavy burdens alone. I'm sure if you met some people from my past, they'd probably say I was "cold... cold-hearted." I wasn't at all. I was just finally emptied.

The price I had to pay, the walls I had to build so high no one was ever there to help me. So I hope that by reading some of my stories, even the smallest parts, someone might understand.

There were countless days I wished upon a star for someone to heal me for someone to simply hold me. Oh, how I wished just to be loved. Don't make the same mistake I did by sticking around for hollow promises that never come true.

My value was never measured by how many people clung to me. I learned to measure the quality and value of those who stayed.

Learning how to forget the ones who forgot you is hard but I learned. The loss of people I thought were true friends turned out to be a gain, because losing them meant leaving behind heartbreak. Keep your circle small. Keep it honest and true. Guard your heart and keep your mind sharp.

One big lesson to learn is that respect is only earned through the balance of trust. Cherish the friendships that are real. Let go of the ones who no longer serve a purpose in your life.

Everyone has been through something that has changed them just as it has happened to me, and to you. Never judge a book by its cover. You never know. I don't like to be judged by anyone. I know for a fact that I am a good person. I will never force someone to be my friend or to see me for who I am. Let people think what they want. I'm okay being misunderstood.

I no longer have the energy to explain my side of the story to those who've already made up their minds about me.

Stop worrying about who's better than you. The truth is you're not in competition with anyone else. The only person you need to be better than is the person you were last year, last month, yesterday. You've grown since last year that's what truly matters at the end of the day. Push your limits and become the best version of yourself.

Whatever you do, don't let other people's success make you feel small. Their journey is not your journey. We all have a story to tell. There have been many days I thought I was broken, but then I realized I'm just a little cracked. Life has handed me some serious shit to deal with, but broken? Never.

Along the way, you'll learn to grow up and realize what's best for you even if it means losing people close to you. Be true to yourself. Be where you need to be for your mental health. Stop begging people to be there for you. Realize that you don't need their attention anymore.

I've learned how to truly not give a damn about people's perception of me. It's better to be alone than to carry the pain and heartbreak of those who weigh on your shoulders.

There's a saying I can't remember where I heard or read it:

"Be the reason someone believes in you not because you're perfect, but because you chose to be kind when you had every reason not to."

I imagine you might be a bit like me you always smile through your storms. You show up with kindness and loyalty in a world that often isn't as kind.

Even today, I walk through life silently, watching a world that keeps trying to break me. I always seem to fall short of being loved, respected, and appreciated. Damn, it always feels like I'm too many steps behind.

Some chapters of my life may seem unreal or untrue, but they are all part of my journey. I keep crossing my fingers, hoping my lessons will finally stop but no such luck yet. Still, there is always hope. Break free of your pain and become aware of *you.*

I learned early that even the smallest victories matter. Those victories were simply getting up, getting out of bed, and moving forward, no matter how heavy my shoulders felt. Keeping one foot in front of the other became my victory each day. My strength grows stronger with every step, and with it comes the power to overcome whatever trauma life throws my way.

Everyone has courage, hope, and the ability to still grow. My success eventually came, but it certainly did not come overnight. Everything takes time, effort, and most importantly belief. Yes, even when things go wrong. Life will always be a challenge to navigate, no matter your age. If you fall a few steps back, the next day you can move three steps forward.

Do not be afraid to make mistakes that's where we learn and grow. We're all human; we all make them. At least you're moving forward on your journey. You're learning how to heal, how to ask, how to tell people *no*. And if "no" doesn't work keep moving, keep learning, and most importantly, keep taking your life back.

Peace is what you need. It's what everyone on Earth needs. But first, you must find that peace within yourself.

Lessons I've Learned Along My Journey

1. You will never control someone's loyalty.

2. You may never be certain they'll treat you with respect and dignity.

3. Just because they mean something to you doesn't mean they feel the same appreciation for you.

4. Some of the people I thought I could trust most in my life were the people I could trust the least.

Inner peace will always be a learning curve a curve built out of trauma. And, holy hell, those "poor me" people do they ever turn things around just to make themselves the victim.

I've had the pleasure a few times in my life of simply watching someone dig their own grave. I'll admit, I've had a huge smile on my face while watching them realize what they've done still pushing their lies right in front of me, thinking I don't have enough brains to figure them out. I just stand back and watch in the darkness. I can see clearly now that my eyes are open.

One day, like me, you'll realize that you are not the weak one at all. You'll see that you were the only one who truly cared.

Slowly, people stop texting. They stop listening. They stop showing up altogether. The silence gets louder and sometimes, the noise is unbearable. Then come the fake apologies from people who don't care. That's when you stop and remind yourself to be strong.

Stop replaying every memory with them. Take a step forward. Maybe put on a song to help guide your mood and remind you of the direction you want to go.

I have to say, as I flip through the social media clutches of life, I've found amazing comfort in listening to **Jelly Roll**. The words in his songs are truly uplifting, to say the least. Some of them helped me articulate the feelings I'd been searching for trying to explain exactly how my heart and soul feel.

Some days, it's even hard to focus. And yes, there will be more days like that as you navigate your new journey of healing and letting go. But now is the time to start standing taller. Start protecting your heart and mind. Your wellbeing depends on it. Healing is about letting go it's about *you* finally learning to love *you*.

Change is hard, but now you know in your heart the strength you need to walk through life not fighting it, but embracing it. Conquer one day at a time. Achieve your goals for today and for tomorrow.

Inner peace will only come from you. Let go of what pain holds you down. Let go of one memory a day. Move forward with the knowledge that you are not alone.

Yesterday, I was out at a restaurant and watched a teen throw a tantrum worse than a child. When the manager arrived, the mother was making excuses, saying, "She's having a bad day her depression got the better of her." But as the mother apologized, the girl was *laughing*.

I was furious. It's bad enough living with real pain and this teenager was using it as an excuse. I was pissed off, yes, I'll admit it. I got up, had my tablet in hand, found the **PTSD** chapter, and approached them. I told the parents to give me five minutes.

The mother started crying fiercely while her husband asked, "What is it?" She kept reading, tears falling harder. When she finished, she handed it back to me, got up, and hugged me.

"That's not the point," I told her. "I don't need your empathy. I and others like me don't need the ignorance of this new generation abusing this condition." I asked her, "How would you feel if you were me?" Her face was covered with shame.

I walked away and finished my lunch. When that family left, the daughter stopped and apologized for her behavior. Unfortunately, there are people who just use that label to gain attention.

Then there are people like me, who took as much pain as possible so someone else didn't have to go through what I did. I would never wish my life on anyone not even my worst enemy. I've watched loved ones do the same thing, and it breaks my heart every single time.

It's a losing battle to call out everyone who abuses or fakes these struggles. It takes too much energy trying.

Each day will bring new meaning to the days that follow. Walk forward with your head held high. *You've got this.*

Yeah, you might fall again and again just as I did but you will come out stronger, more powerful, and more resilient. Finding the new you will bring out the best version of yourself.

It's deeply satisfying to realize you *can* do this and to know you are not alone.

Someone will have your back. Someone will come along and tell you that you are loved, appreciated, and respected that they have unconditional love for who you are, baggage and all.

My baggage became lighter… and so will yours.

Your inner peace will depend on the path you choose for your story this time. Finding peace in your journey is the key. If you know you have toxic people in your life, kick their ass to the curb *now*. The only purpose they will serve is heartache, using you until you have no more purpose for them. Let them go. If you cannot trust them to be there **let them go.**

If they no longer text or email you, except when you're disposable to them, do as they do. Don't reach out. Don't ask them for help. Don't trust them with your loyalty or respect. Believe me when I say this with absolute certainty get their toxic ass out of your life.

Yes, some people will be hard to distance yourself from, but haven't they already done that to you? I don't have all the answers for moving forward, but I've learned more lessons than I ever wanted to.

My biggest fear my deepest belief was embedded in my mind: I truly thought I was supposed to be married with kids. You know, the white picket fence kind of life. That false image life shows you.

I had too many relationships that ended worse than the last. Then, one day decades later I took a massive step out of my book of bullshit knowledge and out of society's expectations of who I was *supposed* to be.

I went from being a housewife, mom, and grandma to realizing too much was attached to a house full of memories both laughter and pain. I changed my business, bought a travel trailer, and started to live alone. I needed to no longer be available a place to crash, a place to be used for what I had.

I went from 1,534 square feet down to 24 feet. By far, letting it all go walking away from being conveniently there to be used was the most freeing decision I ever made.

I found myself, yes, many years later maybe even decades but no one ever told me or showed me how to help myself. There are so many social media apps now, most full of information you don't need. Maybe *you* should start a group to help people. In doing so, walking with someone beside you builds both your strength and your power.

Many hands make light work I didn't have that back in my day. Help someone. Reach out your hand and say, *I can help you.* There's always something that can guide you toward helping yourself.

Find a hobby. Write a book. Write a version of you and your story. Maybe write a poem about how heavy the burden is when you're carrying a broken heart. I used to pour my imagination into creating scrapbooks, and I loved the peace it brought me.

As you continue reading these pages, keep your mind open. Maybe one of my words, one of my experiences, will help you find the part of yourself that finally lets go.

Being alone has become rewarding in ways I never thought possible. I am absolutely okay being alone. I don't need to be in a toxic relationship.

For the last eight years, I've lived on Vancouver Island, and my man lives just below Alaska. We see each other twice a year, both times for two weeks. We talk every day and that's how we both like it. I am never alone knowing he loves me for me, with all my bad habits.

Being alone isn't scary it's not even lonely. I find peace knowing people stopped using me once I could no longer be used for what I had. It's rewarding to know they left my life, and I'm better for it.

Remember: *you* are the only one who can choose to end the toxic relationships in your life. Be brave. Be positive. Be powerful. Take your life back.

When I first started writing, I read *The Secret*. It was a very low time in my life, and someone told me to read it but to read it with an open mind, or I wouldn't understand the message. I laughed. An open mind? Mine was destroyed by depression and emotions so overwhelming they were crippling me.

I read it the first time *without* an open mind. But for days afterward, something kept bugging me in the back of my head. I poured a drink, grabbed my smokes, went outside, and sat down. This time, I had an open mind.

I read it from front to back without putting it down. When I finished, I paused, then reopened it and reread a few pages. For the first time, I understood it's up to me on this journey. It's up to me to change the direction I'm headed in.

That was the day I started writing this book. Now, ten years later, I'm finally finishing it.

After forty years of pain and carrying this heavy burden, the blisters I've gotten from walking this journey have given me life. Unfortunately, the sudden deaths of two beautiful people I loved woke me up. I realized I needed to finish this.

Every day since, I've written even when I thought about starting another book on a different journey. The excitement I've felt these last few weeks has been overwhelming in the best way. Knowing, hoping, praying, and wishing upon the stars that my words might help even one of you with *your* journey fills me with purpose.

Oh my goodness, I seriously had that "now what?" feeling. I had already decided to write more about the fear I've had these past few days. My inner soul feels alive *butterflies swarming through my stomach.*

Now, I have to think again about what's best for me.

I recently read a post on the Jelly Roll fan page it said:

"He reclaimed the stage. He simply reminded everyone what it means to lead with grace, not rage."

In one simple gesture, he changed everyone's mindset about healing and humanity.

Humanity will always be present even for those of us who are broken, trying to mend ourselves along the journey.

Jelly Roll has the perfect song: *"I Am Not Okay."* But it will be okay. That song tells his story of pain and gives you the belief that **you will never be alone.**

As you walk through your story, it's okay to love someone but it's also okay to say goodbye to them. The heartache is real when you lose them because they didn't love you enough. It was hard to find someone who would love me for *me* at the time. I was broken, lost, and emotionally drained. My moods shifted between *"It will be okay"* and *"I can't do this anymore."* It wouldn't get any better.

Life at times seriously felt like emotional whiplash one hour I was hopeful, the next I was spiraling.

Through learning peace, I began to let go. Stop thinking you need to carry the world on your broken shoulders and your aching back. Start with one small thing, then tomorrow do another. On the third day, find peace by letting that memory of heartfelt trauma go.

Most of us who suffer from depression isolate ourselves because, like me, I was always left alone as a child with my emotions. It hurts me now, knowing it still happens.

I still have memories that haunt me the pain I had to endure throughout my life. But I've turned that pain into power. As you can tell, my life has brought me to hell and back more than a few times, but behind closed doors, I still had to show up like nothing was wrong.

I have forgiven many people who have never uttered the words *"I'm sorry."* I've also healed some wounds I still haven't spoken about. Never judge my strength or anyone else's until you've lived through our storms.

You are a truly kind person. Don't let others take advantage of that kindness or your weakness. Remember your value. Know your worth. Learn your value with friends and family. Leave behind the ones who don't support you.

Stop overthinking. Stop chasing. Stop trying to fix things that are breaking you. Stop pouring your heart into people who only take you for granted.

I learned to stop wanting to be chosen by everyone, always pushing my pain down just to keep the peace. It takes a lot not to be angry when you're tired. You *should* be tired tired of the patterns from people who only give you the bare minimum while you give them all of you.

Stop pretending that things are okay when they clearly aren't.

Be done with overthinking. Let people paint you however they want to; they will always label, judge, and twist the story. If your heart is true, your intentions good, and your loyalty unbreakable then that's what matters.

Stand by the people who stand by you. Only choose them if they choose you too. You never need validation for who you are or who you are becoming.

The past will always be the past. The present is the best gift you can give yourself it's the best gift in anyone's life. Be present, because deep down you know tomorrow is never promised. We don't know what will happen tomorrow or next week. That's why living in the present is the biggest gift you'll ever give yourself.

Over the years, I've paid for my mistakes. Karma came knocking on my door more than once. I've lost a lot of friends, and some days it was hard to watch them go. I turned out to be nothing but gossip for some but that became my testimony.

If I hear someone gossiping about me, I say: *"Feel free to talk about who I used to be, about what broke me down. But you'd better invite me to the table so I can show everyone how you let me down when I needed you the most."*

I show with pride how I rebuilt the pieces of my life by myself.

You know what you bring to the table, because they might just bring you back to the fire of hell you fought your way out of. Do not go back to doors you cannot reopen. You are on your way out of anything or anyone trying to stop you.

You are not, and never will be, responsible for anyone's happiness but your own. If they want you to live in their misery, they don't want you to be happy and they shouldn't be in your life.

Never force anyone to choose you. If they think they can find something better than who you are, *let them go.* Do not hold them back. They serve no purpose in your happiness.

Life is way too short to hold on to someone who's not sure they want you. I started to believe in freedom in the truth of feelings instead of pushing them so deep that I could never reach them.

If they must stay, make sure, deep in your heart, they belong on your journey.

Time passes, years go by, and sometimes we find ourselves in the same mental state we were in years ago. Nothing has changed. Nothing has given us a better outlook.

I used to think, *How the hell am I going to get through this heartache this emotional roller coaster with no light at the end of the tunnel?* The only thing I could see was darkness. The only emotion I felt was pain. The only thoughts that ran through my mind were sadness and failure.

I felt like I would never be who I was meant to be. I never thought I was strong enough to prevail.

Oh, have I ever had a thousand inner arguments with myself believing the best in people, even when they were showing me their worst side.

The best have tried me and I'm sure there will be more but now I have the strength, the knowledge, and the power to tell them to **go fuck yourself.**

I know better now.

As time goes by, you learn to watch more and speak less. Sometimes you'll see that when you speak, it falls on deaf ears. People never really listen to me or understand me; they only listen so they can find faults then inflict more pain on my emotional state.

Making mistakes is definitely going to happen. We are human; we are programmed to make mistakes big ones, little ones, even embarrassing ones. My mistakes defined who I was perceived to be growing up. There was no forgiveness.

It took me years to find inner peace. Some days, I wonder if I still have it. At times, I have to look deep down and find it again. It's not easy. No one ever said life was. I have fallen many times in my life. There have been moments when I've thought about the selfish outcome the one that would solve my issues, take my pain away, and stop me from hiding in the darkness. But yet, darkness is the only option for that solution.

Not thinking about it, for me, means facing the inhumanity that people show every day. It's an everyday occurrence. Every day I battle the thought of "no pain, no failure." I win some days, and others I don't. Some days, the thought process and the action all line up it seems we're all lined up to take advantage of that day.

On some days, I wasn't feeling my pain so intensely. As my mind tried to deflect the good day, my grandson my savior walked in and said, "You okay, Nana?" I melted. I got up, just so I could show him that even through my pain, I loved him more than life itself. Since his birth, he has given me more life, more reason, and more drive to get better to take control of it and conquer it.

I definitely haven't conquered all my fears or pain, but my emotional well-being pushes forward, as long as I'm not giving up.

Finding peace will always be a struggle. You will come across other, more painful experiences. You may suddenly feel completely overwhelmed and lost and that's okay. You will get through it. I did.

As I write this about moving forward, forgiving, and letting go, my grandchildren were taken from me because of my narcissistic daughter's complete bullshit. The overwhelming loss, the immense heartbreak it's unbearable.

My daughter knew, with a thousand percent certainty, that taking my time away from those kids would break me emotionally and mentally, especially with my depression. For the last fourteen years, I was their babysitter, sometimes even living with them hands-on, every single day. My grandson loves me. I am *his person.*

After months of not wanting to do anything but lay in bed, I finally got up and told him, "Remember what you want to do when you grow up." He said he wanted to take care of his Nana because I'm going blind.

So I keep his words fresh in my mind. I just have to wait. It is still a struggle losing that unconditional love from my grandkids.

How you handle your emotions is as raw as they may get. Healing won't happen until you choose to stop that horrific cycle of pain and torture. You need to say, *"Enough is finally enough."*

Maybe you can find a new direction in your life. Start by finding a happy spot.

When I write, I bring a book or my tablet and sit by the water sometimes a river, a lake, or the ocean. I use my phone to take pictures of the forest, of children just playing with no cares in the world. Think back to your happy place.

I didn't have a happy place my childhood really sucked ass. But I made it through, even when I thought I wouldn't. I was tested more times than I'm sure ten other people were. But each of us has our own story to tell. Maybe *your* story might help *me*.

There's no right or wrong way to help yourself. There are absolutely no "Books for Dummies" about depression but there's one for everything else in the world.

I certainly don't have the answers to all the questions, but I do have my experience unfortunately, a lot of it. In my day, we didn't have school counsellors; we didn't even discuss anything. I grew up fighting to survive in a world that stripped me of my innocence. But I'm still here just as you are reading this.

There *is* help. You are not alone in this fight, even when you feel overwhelmed by the pain you're suffering and the heavy weight of your burdens. Remember you've got this.

Stand up and say it out loud: **You got this.** 😁

If you lose people along the way, leave them the fuck behind. You do not need to carry the burdens of people who don't respect you or have loyalty to you.

Moving forward in your life, you need to decide on the road you want to travel. Choose *you* this time. Make your journey a story of strength and resilience.

Love yourself for who you are. Don't worry about who loves you. The ones who truly love you unconditionally will still be standing by your side.

Stop chasing people who use you and then throw you to the ground like you're beneath them.

I can't say how many times in my life I dropped the ball. I dropped it simply because I got scared, lost the ability to love myself, and stopped caring about my mental state. Each time I lost my purpose, I fell back into what was "normal" no one loving me, staying in bed, not eating, not communicating.

I fell deeply into that hole. It took forever to climb back out.

Now, you have better access to knowledge from TV, social media, and so many platforms. But have you ever watched them and thought, *Have you really gone through that trauma?* After all, there's a lot of fake news on those platforms.

I'm sure the younger generation focuses a lot on them. Just remember not all information you see is the truth. Either way, I'm glad there's far more help now than there ever was before.

Finding my inner peace was very difficult, as I had suffered enormous trauma from childhood straight through adulthood. As you read my story, you will understand the falling and the getting back up. Even today, or this past month, has been one of the hardest of my life.

I went to work and found my boss naked on the floor colder than I had ever felt from someone. I covered her up. I sat right down beside her, placing my warm hand over her cold one.

My biggest, darkest fear was and still is to die alone. I couldn't leave her just lying there. I felt a calmness wash over my body. I wasn't scared sitting beside her. I made her a promise to finish my book.

I've been going back and forth writing this since 2015, and in just over three weeks, I went from 21,000 words to 60,000. As hard as the memories have been, I still feel I've accomplished something important in my life.

Even years later, I learned how to let it go. I cannot explain the excitement I feel the rush flowing through my blood. I have a man who loves me unconditionally. Yes, he knows all the dark, dirty secrets the good and the bad of my life and he still loves me. Life is ready to change direction when you are ready. Get ready because there is someone out there going through the same thing.

Maybe your inner peace will come to you when you leave a door open, or let down a small piece of the wall you built so high. Sometimes it is extremely hard to get out of our rabbit hole. You need to believe that you deserve to be loved. You deserve to be respected and appreciated. The friends who don't show you at least that much kick their ass to the curb. There are far better people out there who deserve to be part of your life.

Losing some friends becomes a great blessing in disguise. Never chase the ones that leave. Do not chase the ones that use and abuse you. These are not the friends who will help you learn to love yourself, or heal your body, mind, and soul.

It took me three husbands to get it right. I'm not kidding as much as I wish I were. Finding unconditional love isn't easy for some. Keep looking ◑◐, keep changing.

I cry for many reasons for all the ugly thoughts that run through my mind. And when I say "run through my mind," I mean everything in my life: my upsets, my failures, the pressures I cannot overcome. The worst part is hiding my emotions.

I'm far from the only guilty one in this. I have come across so many friends and people even those we know from movies or otherwise who have suffered this deadly, messed-up life of depression. I learned, just like them, how to hide. How not to show the slightest change in who we are.

Hiding has become our greatest accomplishment in life. It has become who we are. We would rather hide the truth than accept it or maybe we just don't know how to deal with it. For the most part, society has swept this disease under the rug. In my day growing up, it was never discussed not even among family.

When I was growing up, I was always told, "That's enough of your damn mood swings." I was told I was begging for attention and in every sense, I was, but not in the way they constantly gave me shit for. I needed help. I knew it, even at a very young age.

But when something isn't relevant in society, it's only chalked up to "mood swings." Oh, how many times I got told to "get a grasp on your PMS." Like that helped. Like that statement still helps today.

Go figure our pain is often caused by the very people who claim to love us.

It has taken me many years to grasp the fact that my mind is not right. My emotions and understanding weren't right either. As I grew older, it became harder. More of life's heartache and trauma entered my life at a rapid pace. The more heartache I suffered, the more depressed and emotional I became.

I became lost in myself. I lost who I wanted to be. I felt hopeless and helpless in every aspect of my life as a daughter, a mother, a wife, a friend, a sister, and even now, as a grandmother. No matter how hard I have tried and continue to try, it will always be the hardest thing to overcome.

Emotions run high in everyone's life but add depression or PTSD to the mix, and it complicates everything. It might feel like it "solves" our inner turmoil, but it only adds a lifetime of heartache to the people who love us.

Can we find inner peace with depression?

Coming from someone who has suffered with both for decades, I would say *yes*.

"Yes" comes with someone supporting you believing in you someone giving you strength from their own achievements and understanding of this damned, infuriating, self-destructive disease.

Always remember: we *can* find inner peace. It will come with kicking the asses of those who don't love you, and keeping the ones who want to help you heal. It takes time to mend a broken heart.

My heart would mend easier if I could see my grandkids, but she's already causing trauma for no reason other than selfishness and cruelty. Oh yes, do I wish I could just slap her. Wrong is wrong and it cannot be forgiven.

Chapter 8: The Anatomy of a Broken Heart

This is when you realize how **fucked up** you really are.

This depends on the day or more importantly, on the realization of how and when your mind, your thoughts, and your body have lost control. But then one may ask, *what is control?*

We all have a different sense of control or a release of stress or, as I would say, my deepest depressive state. There will never be just one. At least not if you're like me, and life just doesn't work that way.

Life, from the start, was supposed to be hard. It was never meant to be easy, never meant to be understood.

I have never understood life. I have seen the difference in happiness I saw that with my own family, with my siblings, and with my cousins, who all seemed to get a much more fulfilled life than I did. Not a "poor me" moment just *it is what it is.*

I was raking the lawn the other day to be exact, the same day my first cousin was being remembered. It was a day I really didn't choose to remember. I personally lost it, for more than one reason or another.

I am on the road with my daughter. I am not sure we can get back from where we are. And yes, of course, it's my fault no matter which way you look at it. I hold my share of responsibility in it.

But at that heartbreaking time, she owned up to her part too. I suppose I understand now but before, no, I did not. Those were *her* actions, not mine. I am heartbroken and barely holding onto the line between surviving and living.

More days are harder than most. The hardest thing to explain to anyone is how alone, how empty, and how low your life can feel that you don't belong, that you don't deserve to be loved.

I did the impossible act over and over again I forgave my daughter. But as I did, I cannot explain the heartache she has given me at the same time.

I knew what being in love looked like. My daughter she was none of it. Not then. But I thank God she may one day find it.

Just as I wish for myself, each and every day that direction of wanting more out of life, more love, more of being wanted and needed. For most of us, it only comes once in a lifetime maybe not even then. Not everyone is that fortunate.

Some people just go out of their way to destroy you and me.

Make sure you tell them to aim well, because if by chance they miss, I will, with certainty, exclude them from my life.

It's time to let go of those who disappoint you.

Remember one thing: most people only talk to you when they *want* something or *need* something.

Learn to only respond when you are completely bored.

At times when I said, "I hated you," I hated myself more for letting you hurt me over and over again.

I just won't miss you anymore.

I have accepted so many things over the years that I will never accept again. You can leave people out of your life simply by closing the door and finally walking away.

Walking away will one day be the best thing you ever do for yourself.

Do not let those who used you those who caused you deep pain ever back into your heart.

They don't deserve to return when *they* decide they want to.

Love whether from family or friends can help you through your darkest times. You have changed because of them, but now you have changed enough to open your eyes *to* them.

Learning to trust takes time. Do not jump to it too quickly that would be a big mistake.

I've learned not to be in "fighting mode" anymore. I simply have no desire to argue with anyone.

I learned to just walk away to seek inner peace, both mentally and spiritually.

Back in the early days, I spent way too much energy being resentful, angry, and lost. Now I've learned there are just some people I prefer never to be in contact with.

Placing them *outside your walls* is the best place for them.

Your strength is not built by everything in life going right. Strength is built by the hits you've taken the hard ones and still refusing to stay down.

All those broken moments, all those tough days that's where your strength is built.

In the silence of your many battles, that's where your power is born.

After you fall, rise again. Each time you get back up, you prove that nothing and nobody can break you now unless you give them back their power.

Do not allow that.

One of the best things I've learned so far is how to enjoy my life, even amid the storms. As long as I'm alive, there will always be problems that's just life.

There will still be chaotic days but you can always find a way to smile, to find peace and happiness through it all.

We all need moments of solitude a space to reflect on our thoughts and emotions without distraction. It's about reconnecting with yourself, understanding what you truly need and want life to be.

Your emotional breaks are essential for your wellbeing. They give you the chance to regain balance and restore your energy.

Giving yourself time to breathe and believe is essential. It gives you purpose and a clearer perspective.

It is *never* selfish to prioritize your mental and emotional health and wellbeing.

Always remember: it's important to be the best version of yourself you can be.

I know my worth after decades and I will never again beg for anyone's attention or validation.

I am past that.

I will absolutely never be someone's backup plan.

And so many times in my life, I have felt this truth deep within my inner core.

If you have found someone who knows your value who understands *the whole you,* depression and all and they stand just as tall as you, then I hope you have found your person.

Remember, if you're just searching to pass time or playing games, you may regret what you might have missed. I say this because I was young, I was dumb, and I certainly took life for granted.

Part of maturity is realizing you don't need to be around drama. Start choosing calm over stress. Put distance between yourself and the people who disrespect you. Start prioritizing your peace, your mental health, and your happiness above everything else.

Always remember the old saying: *You cannot force a cheater to be loyal, you cannot twist a bad friend into being a good one, and you certainly cannot make a liar find their moral compass.*

We need to stop spending time with people who do not make us feel good the ones who, without thinking, stab us directly in the back.

At some point, you must stop giving second chances when no one ever gave you a first.

It takes days to recover from overhearing a conversation where someone calls you small, broken, and unworthy. Stop convincing yourself they're not all bad. You just need to find the true ones.

Silverstone once said in a podcast, *"Let them talk. Let them judge. Let them spin the stories about you they've heard. Let them count you out as an outsider. You are not misleading your purpose, and don't doubt your path. Why? Because to truly succeed, you must be willing to endure the negativity that comes with it."*

I don't even know how to explain what I'm feeling anymore.

Every day, it feels like a constant storm inside me. It's hard to find the words to describe it all I've ever known is that I hurt.

I hurt emotionally, physically, and mentally.

At times, the silence becomes something I cannot hide. It's never just one thing. Some days it's the constant disappointment the fake-ass smiles I endure every day, the feeling of being forgotten, even when surrounded by people.

Some days I want to talk; other days, I just want to disappear quietly so no one has to see me struggling as I cry in silence wiping my tears again and again.

So many days are like this. Some days bring laughter, others only emptiness.

I always say I'm fine, but just like you I'm not.

Let people ghost you. Let them betray you. Let them run their mouths about you.

This is your opportunity to see their true colours by giving them all the freedom in the world to be exactly who they are and in that process, you find out who *you* are.

I certainly don't have time to hate anyone while I'm busy building myself back up.

I either love you, or I don't. There's no in-between.

I don't strive to be everyone's friend.

Things will be hard there will be setbacks. People will doubt you. But here's the truth: their doubts mean absolutely nothing. Your belief means everything.

We only get one shot at life so start living it.

You have dreams, right? Don't we all?

Then you need to act like it. Stop waiting for the perfect moment there might never be one.

There is no perfect moment. The moment is *now*.

You're not too young. You're never too late. You may feel broken, but you are exactly where you need to be.

It's up to you to start building the life you've dreamed of.

It's been a hard week for me but even harder for my aunty and uncle.

My cousin… it was the first time our family lost one of us out of order. We had always gone in life's order: first Grandpa, then Grandma, then my mom. But a cousin? That's not who we should've said goodbye to.

I sit here right now thinking it should have been me first.

My kids are grown. I had the chance to be a Nana and watch my children grow.

I've never been loved by my family not by my siblings, not by my daughters.

My cousin had her whole life ahead of her. Mine feels done.

My goodbye would be just like my mother's nothing more than a short of vodka to say farewell.

There are so many days I wish I could go back and have a different conversation with my cousin that day. I'm not sure it would have made a difference, but I like to think it might have.

She always struggled with how our family behaves when we make mistakes.

Fuck the grudge is forever. They'll remind you of it constantly. Forgiveness was never part of the family except for one aunty and one uncle.

The disgrace you feel when family gathers the unwanted feeling is so strong you could cut it with a knife.

I don't just show up at any family member's house, not for anything.

I even live just blocks away from my aunty, her family, and cousins all here in the same town.

In two years, not a single visit.

I've known since I moved here that my aunty knew, but black sheep don't get reached out to.

When you feel uncomfortable and unwanted, you simply lose the desire to visit.

Life with depression is hard enough we don't need our own family adding to that stress.

My only regret would be not seeing my one aunty and one uncle the two who forgave all us cousins for making mistakes.

Damn, we were kids. Some of us were angels. Some of us not so much, like me.

Outcast until the day I die.

How sad to think that when you die, you'll be alone when you take your last breath, when you smoke your last joint… what then?

I don't want a new life after this one. I want my journey to end.

If you're wondering as you read this yes, I do believe in reincarnation.

Through my life, I can say with certainty that I drowned in a previous one. I've had a fear of water my entire life the constant feeling of drowning.

I never went into lakes or rivers unless I could stand in them. I will not and absolutely have not done diving or swimming in deep water.

I have to say, even now at my age, people do not excite me anymore. If absolutely no one talks to me, it seriously doesn't bother me at all. I certainly don't have the energy to argue or give my time to certain people who have nothing good to say. With my current state of growth, I've learned that if I need to be alone I'll go with it.

State of mind is always going to be essential to everyone. Finding that peace can be challenging, but believe in yourself. Believe that you've gone through enough to finally have some control.

Over time, I've learned how to hide the noises. People think I'm so strong, but the real truth is I'm not. I may be just as tired as you are. I'm tired of carrying pain I can't explain. I'm tired and yet I always act like I'm not.

I've found that when I want something, I work hard and go for it. Does it work every time? Absolutely not. But I move forward and continue to try. I've learned not to depend on anyone but that doesn't mean you can't. I just never came across someone who loved me enough to truly care. Fuck, still waiting on that one. Isn't that sad? That feeling always brings me back to my cousin the pain

I felt, and the thoughts that maybe I should've said something different.

I realized that if I wanted something, I had to work twice as hard as most people. I found early in life that I could achieve anything well, to a point. I put one foot forward whenever I had the chance. But chances for me were few and far between.

My thought around my life back then was this: I didn't depend on anyone then, and I don't think I do now. That's a sad statement to make especially when all I ever wanted was to help others move forward.

Right now, I feel like I need a break from everyone and everything. Life has been overwhelming lately. I feel like I'm constantly running on empty. The daily grind, the endless responsibilities, the constant noise of the world it's all taken its toll. And you know what? If you really want to talk shit about me, go ahead. I finally don't give a shit.

My intuition has always told me that I've fought every one of my journeys alone. I've fought to live through every moment, but as life goes I'll die alone. Dying alone doesn't bother me like it used to when I was younger. Now, it's just the way life is going to be.

I feel extremely bad for my grandkids, always having their lives filled with bullshit from their narcissistic mothers.

A few times over the years, my little sister has mentioned an incident from when she was a young child. When we talked about it, she was so full of anger and hatred. I'd heard about that incident back when I was in Grade Nine when it happened. She never knew, nor heard about, my aggressive reaction how I snapped on the boy, or should I say "man," who touched her. I beat him senseless. I broke his nose.

To this day, my sister knows nothing about that. Funny thing the kids who knew why I lost it that day staged a full-on student walkout. We even made the news. Promises were made that nothing would ever be said about the roller-skating incident, where my sister was stripped of her innocence her belief that no bad people lived around us.

To this day, I have never forgiven or forgotten that moment. Unfortunately, my sister has always felt like I let her down but it was completely the opposite.

Growing up, I seriously prayed to get any of the family genetics the cervical cancer, or any of the other family illnesses. But I truly prayed that I'd get them. I prayed because I was the black sheep. I prayed because no one loved me not then, maybe not ever.

I always sat on the sidelines. Fuck, they would talk about issues meant to be secret, and not a single person realized I was there. No one noticed me for years. They shared the family secrets with other people I knew. I heard the stories I just never heard the ones about me.

Even as I write my story, I still feel anger. Holy fuck, people even your kids made mistakes, but I wasn't allowed to.

It took decades before I found out why my so-called godmother hated me so much. Why the fuck wouldn't you, as an adult, say something sooner? For decades, nothing. I found out during my sister's disgust toward me when our grandmother passed away.

That time with my sister, when she drove me home after our grandmother's funeral, will be something I will never forget in my lifetime the pain, the disturbing tone, the pure anger in her voice, and the silence that said, *I will never love you again.*

From that day forward, it took about three months before I came out of that extremely deep depression.

As if that emotional experience wasn't enough on the way back, as I brought my sister to my auntie's, she just unleashed on my kid. Holy fuck, like who gave you the right to do that? Who gave you that right?

To this day, I am still pissed off about it. When our mother died, we hugged for a brief second and said "peace" while standing at my uncle's place. Still, oh, the anger that lives inside me to this day.

It's almost like she's angry that I wasn't there when she was truly sick maybe a few times, but if you're not going to say anything and just hold it over someone's head, that's on you.

I felt bad, but also angry. I had cancer twice both times completely on my own, taking care of my small children after serious surgery. She had everyone, while I had no one.

I really didn't expect a soul to be by my side I knew deep down that not a single one would be. I knew then that the love my family had for me was slim to none, even today.

Our mother passed last year, and I haven't had a single word from my sister since just the occasional birthday or Christmas "hello." Growing up, they always talked badly about our mother, and yet in the end, it was all my fault.

Holy hell, okay… but her choice to disown me? Yeah, granted, I caught her off guard, but for years my siblings said over and over again how Mom screwed over Dad.

I had first-hand knowledge of my mother screwing our dad over. I was the same age they were when they split up. I felt that I had to start over after my second marriage well, why the hell couldn't she? Always stoned on pills.

But this time, I felt for my father. I thought maybe, after fifteen years, he might finally love me because I gave a statement to stop the unfair treatment my mother was giving him. I stood up. That choice cost me the next eighteen years without my mother.

Would I do it again? I would have to say yes. It wasn't my father's fault for the breakdown of their marriage. At some point, she should have just taken responsibility for her own actions. Saying that still sends shivers down my spine, even today decades later.

I can remember the day it all started to go really bad with our parents. Of course, the other kids had too much positivity in their lives. My dad kept questioning my mom about her shifts at work. My mom, at the time, was the head RN at the hospital.

Well, my mom decided to start taking the medication meant for dying patients. My dad, nevertheless, didn't believe her excuses. She was abusing the system and he knew it. So did I. Man, I hated having my room right beside theirs. I heard way too much as a kid. Those words, those fights I can never unhear them.

The trials and tribulations you go through are unbelievable at times. They become the hardest part of understanding what you're about to encounter experiences like no other. I have never, nor will I ever, say depression is easy. It's solely up to you to find ways to handle the emotions and figure out the mental part. Both will test you and make you question yourself.

You've grown. You've become very strong. Moving forward with calm and ease is how you handle yourself from here. Move forward knowing you have overcome the worst life can throw your way. Remember, you now have the ability to stand tall. You are strong, you will succeed, and you will survive.

At times in life, you need to take a step back take a deep breath and refocus on yourself and your well-being. Finding peace sometimes takes a little time. Remember, time will heal and give you the chance to move forward. Someday, take one baby step. Maybe the next day, double that size. Life is worth taking steps forward, no matter what stands in front of you.

No matter what life throws at you, take a deep breath, then choose your path A or B and go down that road to change what you need to. Address what bothers you. Take hold of what makes you distressed. Own it and then let it go. Rehashing the past only makes moving forward more difficult and emotionally challenging, both physically and mentally. If you don't get a handle on it, it can destroy everything you've built, everything you've changed, everything that's made you the new you.

Dealing with your children after they become adults is trickier than anyone tells you. My girls have caused me so much drama and devastating trauma. Sad to say, they seemed to enjoy causing havoc in everyone's lives even causing trauma to their own children.

My grandson is a good example of the damage a bad mother a narcissistic mother can inflict on her children for her own gain.

Over the years, I've listened to my own girls talk badly about me. I've listened for years to their lies. Some made me shake my head so hard I thought it would fall off. Both only care about what they get out of the picture. I've never seen either of them regret what they've done or said not once. They drive the gossip further and push the complete negative version of me.

The result of taking my grandkid from me was devastating not just emotionally, but physically and mentally. Still, I forgave. I allowed them to continue with their bad behavior until one day, I didn't. I haven't talked to my youngest child in over eight years.

I miss the child she used to be, but I don't waste my time. My mental well-being is more important. But saying that, I still haven't seen my granddaughter since. Oh, I really miss her. The regret of not being able to watch her grow has been traumatic for me.

It's been traumatic because I watched my daughter not give a shit about her own child. When she was young, she always said she didn't want to be a mother. Yet, she purposely trapped a guy with a pregnancy. My heart has hurt for many years from the damage she caused purposely and she never thought twice.

I had to make a decision to let go. My mental health was collapsing right in front of me. I had to let go. I will forever miss them, but maybe when my granddaughter is old enough, I'll see her again.

The older daughter holy fuck that's a completely over-the-top narcissist. Through thick and thin, I kept forgiving her. I've never heard more devastating bullshit from another human and it came from my own child.

Twice she has taken her kids from me, based solely on me being her mother. Believe me, I learned early with my children that sometimes you have to put them in their place. Doing the right thing cost me everything.

When you become a parent, you are their parent until the day you die. I've never cared what people thought of me when I put my kids in their place. I tried so hard not to raise them to be selfish, narcissistic, or completely disrespectful. But this time there is no forgiveness for my daughter. This time was absolutely the last time.

Watching her put her ex under the spotlight of Child Protective Services lying through her teeth, lying so badly to the courts was unbearable. The courts here have let my grandkids down. As far as I've seen, nothing's changed. There have been way too many second chances, too many heartbreaks, too many lies, and too much willful, malicious harm done all at the expense of the kids.

My opinion of people who behave in such a malicious way? They should be ashamed of themselves. They should hang their heads in shame but they don't. For some dumb reason, judges always believe the mother. Absolutely fuck that. She's callous and always will be.

I only hope one day the kids can heal from this from the true heartache, the real menace of pain.

This is why I walked away. Not everyone is worth fighting for. If there's consistency in bad behavior and constant pain let go and walk away. Then you'll have control.

Watching malicious people do horrific things breaks something deep inside you. It makes you question everything you know. Life is hard absolutely but it doesn't need to be harder because of the ones you love. The heartache will only end when the behavior changes. Until then, I will spend my days worrying about them every single moment of every single day.

My one wish is that they come through this with as little damage as possible but knowing my daughter, that's unlikely. I will always believe that, as a parent, we have the right to tell our kids when they are doing wrong. We have a duty to correct their behavior, especially when other lives are being seriously affected. Having a calm, relaxed attitude teaches them nothing. Be the one who stands up for that child you see suffering.

Become that person when you see something, you say something. When you see bad behavior or someone being traumatized, **step the fuck up and help**. Stop letting pain and suffering be allowed. Stop the traumatic madness.

I've been staring at my tablet for half an hour trying to find a way to decompress. The anger I had so deep inside me today took me for a loop. As good of a person as I try to be, I remember that hating someone takes way more energy than your soul or wellness can afford. But I cannot shake it. Literally, my blood is boiling and breaking at the same time.

Today we had a **celebration of life** for my friend and also my boss. While my employment there wasn't very long, I loved her attitude and who she showed herself to be: a genuine person with a loving heart. I quickly became the delivery driver as well as the market girl *lol*. Meeting the people she knew gave me such awe, such a warm feeling of love. Something I wish I had, even for just a single day.

One morning, I went in as usual, checking the temperatures, and noticed our main freezer wasn't working and yes, it was full of products. For the four months I worked there, it was mostly fun but also full of intoxicating drama, in abundance. When her mouth opened, I'd cringe. I quickly became angry, as this one employee would bash the boss, bash the house, bash the business and, more importantly, bash *her*.

Oh, fuck, daily was I angry. I said a hundred times, "Enough!" We had plenty of heated fights at work, for sure. In the end, someone who was so spiteful a true narcissist showed me what dishonesty and cruelty really looked like. I have never in my life felt such disgrace for another person's lack of respect.

I had this drive in me to protect my friend, yet every chance this other person got, she pounced on her. She berated her every single day, breaking her down with words like, "Your past you need to deal with it now. Your life is this way because of you." That's just some of the things she said.

Then came the day I found my friend my boss deceased. Naked. Cold. On her bedroom floor, reaching for the door. I placed a blanket over her body and sat down beside her. I waited with her until the others arrived. As I sat there, I took a deep breath, placed my hand over hers, and just talked. I told her I completely understood that I was with her.

For some reason, I felt her presence as I sat holding her hand. The room was warm, and the birds outside were singing so loudly. There were many moments that brought me great joy in knowing her, but I didn't want her to say goodbye alone.

As I started whispering, "It's okay. Go fly high," the impression of hands pressed down on the blanket. I felt peace true peace being there in that moment.

And from this experience, she gave me two important things no one ever had before. About a week before her death, there was an incident with the van and a freezer holy shit, my bad and the guilt I felt was overwhelming. She walked over and hugged me.

I had never been hugged like that before not by many souls in my entire life. That single hug she gave me was a simple, powerful feeling I had waited fifty-four years to experience. OMG, I will never forget those two precious memories with her.

The daily pain and heartache I felt from that other employee turned into anger. But as I grew to know my boss better, my compassion for her deepened, and my anger toward the other one grew stronger.

One day I had enough. Weeks before my boss fell ill, the lies and harsh misconceptions this other woman spread to other employees were just too much. Her cruelty caused real harm emotional, spiritual, and mental harm not to mention the toll it took on my boss's appetite and health.

I was upfront when asked, and I didn't lie.

Being the noble person the one with true loyalty you can still lose yourself. Be careful who you trust. Be even more careful who you're loyal to. If someone tells you once that another person has bad intentions for you, that they only want something from you and will never give anything back remember, evil is just that. They present themselves as true, but they're wolves in sheep's clothing.

You'll find, throughout life, you have different breaking points and some will be more powerful than others. Over time, I've learned to use my voice. Life has taught me to be *that one* the one who finally speaks up, who finally takes hold of who they want to be.

So, speaking up got me absolutely nothing except kicked to the curb when my friend, my boss, passed away, and the evil woman had me dismissed.

So today was the celebration. Even hours later, my blood is still boiling because the people who need to see her true colors are blindsided by the false light. I try very hard every day to be a good person I help when I can, I give when I can, and I am present when I am needed. But sometimes, you still lose that battle between good and evil. If anything, you'll always have days when you need to stop, rethink, and regroup.

Although my heart still aches for my friend my loss because it was way too soon, I also know, from the times we talked, that depression kills in more ways than one. My lesson from all this has taught me that I really need to find an outlet to release my anger, to let go of the deep negative thoughts that imprint on my mind.

Yes, even today as I write this, and probably when you're reading it, I will still come across good days and bad days. But now, you have so much more information than I ever had. Use what you learn to help guide you, to bring yourself to a sense of peace. Life will always move forward you just need to start your journey too.

Oh yeah, make no mistake life is definitely going to get fucken hard. Maybe for some, it's easier. But when you finally have the tools, the knowledge, and someone who loves you, you have what you need. Take a step each day. Maybe tomorrow it'll feel like two steps back, but you're still moving forward. With each new day comes a new start.

The only one who can really change you make that day be *today*. The world wasn't built in a day, so it will take more than a few days to change the direction your life is going. The path you take can always shift toward a better, life-saving direction. It will always be up to you which way you go. No one can force your hand, and no one can tell you what to do.

Living with depression is a lifelong struggle, but it doesn't always have to be. We learn and we grow from every experience. Standing on your own will come you'll learn to strive for what's best for you and for your wellbeing. Life isn't easy whatsoever, but it can be handled.

Over time, memories will fade. The weight of the world won't feel as heavy. Day by day, your heart will start to feel more love than loss. The most important lesson we can ever learn is to let go let go of what hurts, of what causes heartbreak. Letting go of those people, well... some of them, that's going to be one of the hardest things you'll ever do. But you *will* come out the other side, and you *will* overcome your fears.

You'll be able to overcome I say that with certainty, even today. Not only did I find and lose a friend a few weeks ago, but I was also losing another at the same time to brain cancer. I'm not sure I can find the right words to describe the feeling the anxiety, the deep pain every time I opened Facebook.

This friend... oh man, she was one of the greatest souls I ever met. True, loving, giving, spiritual, with an amazing heart. This beautiful soul I met almost fourteen years ago in Victoria. The day I met her, I knew she and I would be friends forever or so I thought.

One of the very first things Jo and I talked about was DNRs. My health wasn't good at the time, and she shared one of her own concerns she had a tumor in her brain. Of course, I asked about surgery and all that, but she didn't want to impact the quality of life she had. She never knew how long she'd have, but when we met and became friends, it changed both our lives.

Oh, her artistic talent was amazing. After a few years of distance because we both moved I went to see her after I found out the tumor had metastasized and ripped her life right out from under her. I always knew about her DNR, and so did her parents. But out of pure selfishness, they didn't honor her wishes.

So, for eight excruciating months of her not being herself, I watched the days crawl by. As more months passed, then weeks, maybe even days left, my anxiety had never been tested so deeply. Each day I woke up with fear, pain, and heartbreak. Every time I wanted to check Facebook, my gut twisted terrified I'd see the post that she was gone. Thank God she was alive... but truly, at what cost? And who suffered more?

This ache hasn't gone away not a day since I saw her on her wedding day. I brought her something borrowed, something blue, and her veil. I was so proud of her moment becoming a wife but my heart broke. It came at the cost of her deepest wish not to be left like she was. The pain in her eyes when we met in that hospital room I'll never forget it.

She couldn't walk down the aisle. She couldn't dress herself. Most importantly, she had lost who she was that vibrant, beautiful woman. Her mental health and wellbeing weren't meant to take the journey she was forced into. That hurts. But now, I am at peace she's at peace. My pain is gone with her.

The loss of two very special people in just two weeks was, to be honest, fucken hard emotionally, physically, and mentally.

Not being heard will always be one of my downfalls. I told lies when I was young just like any kid but I grew up. I got over it. People who pretend and lie don't have your back. Their intentions and integrity are not true to you.

Step away. Bring happiness. Bring peace. Then you will find love.

Somewhere along your journey, you will start to learn not only how to judge people, but also how to watch their body language because that tells the true story. If someone stabs you in the back upon meeting you, then that person well, kick them the fuck out of your life. Anyone who stabs you in the back once will do it a thousand times if you let them get away with it the first time.

People's perspectives can be tentative because of someone else's lies, and I lost the chance to help with something personal something my heart needed to heal. But because of one single person, I lost that time.

Before I go back and read this, I can bet there are a few times where I either repeated myself or maybe forgot something that needed to be said. There are a million and one things out there to help any person cope but cope with what? Are you going in the direction your life needs to go? Do you have a support system? Or have you finally just let…the fuck go?

Life will move forward only when you take the steps to let go to stand up for yourself. Make the decision that *you* and your wellbeing matter.

Yes, you read that correctly I did have a meltdown. I had a loss of emotional control. Every now and then, that will happen. Take your time to deal with it. Take your time to process the pain. My pain and the torture I gave myself weren't good still aren't. Learning how to cope will always surprise me, as it should for you too.

As you've read, these last few weeks have tested me for sure emotionally, physically, and spiritually. But they also gave me the drive to finally continue with my writing, to tell my story in hopes that I can help just one person. My journey was far from easy. Some things, I suppose, were just brought on by the life I was living at the time.

In all the years it has taken to get this far, I have written more in the last three weeks than I did in all the earlier years of trying to kick depression's ass. These last two weeks have opened my eyes, yet broken my heart. More importantly, they've allowed me to open up about what life is right now.

No, I don't think my heartache can ever be completely mended. But I can walk through life now trying to mend the broken lines of love. Time, life, lessons, and memories will one day bring some peace into your life. You can always forgive to release the pain no one ever said you had to forget.

You might find, as I did, that forgetting someone's actions is easier said than done. We may forget what they did, but the *words* the words burn into our minds. The date, the time, the moment those we never forget. It's far easier on many people, even those with PTSD, to handle physical pain than mental. I got beat plenty of times over my life.

I cannot remember every day it happened, but the days I was mentally abused will forever be remembered every detail burned into memory. And oh, how I would love to punch the living shit out of my so-called friend. What a piece of work... cruel. A person I truly hate. I don't even hate my first husband for raping me so that definitely says something about who this cunt is.

For the first time, I feel knocked completely off my feet. I've truly felt the pain of having absolutely no love, no empathy, nothing. I found the most selfish human possible.

Even standing stronger than I was years ago, you still fall down. When your shields are down and you let someone in and they destroy you emotionally, mentally, and physically your body loses control. That day, mine did. But I've been forcing my anger into my story, and yes, it's been helpful. More importantly, we are human we're going to make mistakes. What matters is how we learn and how we get to a better place.

There have been many times when, even surrounded by people, I still felt lonely. That loneliness was definitely worse because real loneliness is never about the absence of people it's about the absence of understanding.

I learned to stop wanting people's company. As life went on, I started to crave something deeper a personal connection. It's far more important to find the soul who sees you for *who you are.* You'll start to see who you truly are and the version of yourself you're becoming.

It's better to have one person who has your back unconditionally emotionally, physically, spiritually who stands by you even with your faults. The others mean absolutely nothing. They will never see the true you because they don't believe in you. They don't have loyalty or respect. So leave them behind. You will meet people, as I have, who see beyond the mask you've worn for so long.

I never knew at first that my loneliness would prepare me for so many cold, hard days filled with pain and trauma. But it gave me practice for what was right in front of me. I've had people ruin my peace by telling me what others were saying about me. Here's what you say back: *What they said about me? Keep that shit to yourself. They told you, not me so seriously, go fuck yourself.* Keep your peace.

Life is way too short to listen to shit like that. You need to decide if the pain or the person is worth it. Life isn't going to care how tired you are of the pain or heartbreak step forward today and own it. Let it go.

Over the years, I've thought of a few ways to let things go. Write down your worries, fears, and memories. Put them in a bottle and release it. Blow up some balloons, send out positive thoughts inside, and let them go.

I may even include the last recorded message she sent me how just plain heartless and shameful her behavior was. The level of disrespect was beyond anything I've seen. Because of the actions of one single piece of shit, the celebration of my friend's life was a complete bomb. I have a pain in my heart that the people who meant the most to her didn't have the guts to say goodbye. Yup… sorry, still angry but things are a process.

I may just have to add a few more chapters. With this last few years of shit, I could probably add two or three more. *LOL.*

Chapter 9:
Navigating the Storm: Loss, Anger, and Glimmer of Peace

I'm sitting here chuckling to myself, trying to heal from this nightmare this trauma. I lost control. I lost my sense of being strong, of knowing better than to fall down the rabbit hole. I knew better, but life didn't make it easy for anyone to see what was truly happening. The truth was so far away, it was breaking me.

Being broken has happened so many times in my life that it almost feels normal. Well, it *used to* but now I know better. Now I know that, for the most part, my time and energy are just being used by those who claim to love me, to need me. Like right now, I feel unwanted, unneeded, and certainly not valued in any way possible. I was more than what I was ever given credit for. I meant more to her, and just because of one single person, I lost a special moment the chance to be there at her end.

You will certainly come across friends in your life whether at work, a bar, or on social media the ones who demand all your time because it's always about *me… me… me*. Run. And fucken run fast. Those are the ones who will, without a second thought, stab you in the back. They'll take your good name down just to save their own.

They will, at any cost, keep you at a distance so you can't expose their true selves. A narcissist will always make others look bad, and they'll do it at any cost. People who lie about you, who tell untrue stories about your life people who show no integrity, no respect, not even the simplest loyalty they are not meant to be in your life. The only thing I can say with absolute confidence is that they will only break you down. They will make everyone around you believe their lies. The truth won't matter when people are fooled by deceit.

My goodness, my blood is still boiling over. Sometimes, I guess, you just need to step back and take more than one deep breath. Having this much anger built up is not a good thing. It's given me headaches, loss of appetite, lack of sleep, and most importantly, it's taken control of my emotional, mental state and wellbeing. I'm smart enough to know she used who I am the good person I am against me.

For decades, I've kept my distance from drama. Drama only meant more problems, more anxiety. I know my back broke fighting two people who tried to damage my integrity, my values, and the morals of who I've become over these last few decades.

My daughter well, I guess I shouldn't even say "for" as my eldest daughter has bashed me her entire life, blaming me for her shortcomings. Fuck no. I made my kids own their actions back then. I didn't want them to face the same heartaches I did. My daughter talked about everyone and always behind their backs. People finally started to notice, and now she really doesn't have any real friends.

Between my daughter taking the kids away and cutting off all contact with me through her direct, malicious lies, she got exactly what she wanted. I have to say the system is very much broken, especially if you're a man wanting custody of your kids. You live here? Good luck. I saw red in that courtroom red like I've never seen before. My kid shouldn't have been granted full custody, and that's on the judge that day. How incredibly unjust you were. Not to me, but to the wellbeing of the children and the relationship they had with me. That judge should have been required to take a parenting class and learn what family unity really means.

There will be plenty of lessons about making the wrong friends. It's in our nature to want to believe in someone's honesty and loyalty. Once in a while, though, take a step back and make people *earn* your trust show that they'll be there for you no matter what.

But if this person is using you solely for personal gain, put on your shoes and walk the fuck away. Don't wait to be hurt you may not survive the heartbreak again.

Take it from someone who has lived it and is still living it. You never need a big group of friends. You just need one or two who help you grow, who lend you a hand when you need it, instead of walking away when you need them the most. Living life without the hand of someone who loves you unconditionally is difficult it's hard, it's lonely. Sometimes, the silence of our pain and the burden of the world on our shoulders gets heavy.

Go back to the beginning of my book and read the quotes I left in those chapters. Finding peace and love can be challenging, to say the least but it's out there for all of us to find.

First, find yourself. Then, give yourself permission to start healing. You have to love *you*, even if no one else does. Being broken doesn't mean you can't live life being broken just means you need time to heal those parts of your story. Talking about your story is a good place to start.

That's how I started my journey how I took the first of many steps forward. Even when I fell down, I got back up. I tried again and again. But one day, I did it. I made it through a tough transition from hating myself to loving myself, even when no one else did.

Everyone's story is different. The challenges aren't necessarily the same. Some trauma cannot be forgotten it lies too deep within us. As I moved through my story, I was beaten along the way. I was beaten physically, emotionally, and mentally throughout my life.

If you were to ask me even today decades after my helpless life began I would say I'd take the physical beating every single time over the mental and emotional abuse. It's easier to forget how you got that black eye, how you broke your arm in two places, how beaten and bloody you were. I would still take the beating.

My emotional and mental health took a different path in my brain. The hitting always went away yeah, of course it pissed me off, and yes, it made something inside me change. But I was always coherent enough to forgive that kind of abuse. The mental part though the emotional words that dig into the deepest parts of your being those stay. They keep talking in your head.

I can still remember the words of my first husband. I was five feet tall, maybe a hundred pounds, with huge tits, and he said, *"I don't find you attractive. I don't like the way your body looks and feels after the kids."* He constantly tried to berate me all day, every day.

You see, those words stay. That image sits right at the front of my memories. It never goes away. We can always forgive, and we should but at the same time, be careful about who you let back into your life. Words will always stay with us. Words, when spoken, bring our memories back. Talking can heal us but when used by the wrong people, words hurt even more than the last person you let into your life.

Wanting to have friends, to be part of a family, is something that's etched into all of us. It's human nature to want to belong, to be part of something. But you need to find that *something special* you're looking for in your love life, your work life, and your life overall. Just because you were born into a family doesn't necessarily make them family.

For decades, I've had little to do with mine. They never loved me before even as a child so I give them no reason to hurt me now. As hard as it was, I learned that I didn't need love all the time. I needed to love myself first for my destiny, for my wellbeing.

It's definitely out there, don't get me wrong. Lots of people have amazing luck with family, friends, jobs, and life. But not all of us get that kind of opportunity not until we stand up and say, *"It's my turn. I got this.* " Stand tall, take a deep breath, and move forward into the change you want to see the change that is your only option and your best opportunity.

As you read this, remember: all our lives are different. Trauma might never look the same, but one day, by chance, you might meet someone just like you. Reach your hand out and they'll reach back. Take hold of changing yourself into the person you want to be. It's all up to you. Finding peace is worth searching for. Find peace to forgive, peace to let go, and strength to move forward.

Since I began writing this book, I've made it a point to practice what I'm saying. I'm still working on things I need to let go of. I always try to find peace within heartbreak because having peace is part of letting go of what hurt you. It doesn't mean you have to forget. At some point, we all need to let go of the pains from our past maybe even some from our future too.

All my writing over these last three weeks was triggered by a traumatic experience. In a split second, I lost the one person who held me like it mattered and then it was gone. I felt robbed. I felt heartbreak like never before. Then, the loss of another friend right after was too much for me to bear.

My heart aches for both of my friends both taken in tragic circumstances. Both heartbroken. Both gone too soon. Both were women who could walk into a room and roar, whose energy and spirit filled every space. They'll forever live on in the hearts of those blessed to have known them.

Both would have given you the shirt off their back. They'd lift their hands to help you through your pain. They'd simply hug you and say, *"I love you,"* and you knew they meant every word. I'm going to miss those two more than words can say. The world lost two people who gave so much to everyone else.

I have to touch on the guilt that consumes you. Remember when I said the mental part is sometimes harder to deal with? Well, my younger friend always knew she had a brain tumor but chose not to have surgery. There was no guarantee she'd be cured or even be able to walk or talk again. She chose to live to love life and be present. Oh, how I loved that spirit in her.

The day I went to see her get married, after the tumor had grown, she'd already had brain surgery, suffered a stroke, and lost the use of her right side. Her memories and speech had to be relearned. She couldn't really feed herself. She always stated firmly, *"DNR."* I knew it. Her parents knew it. If I knew they knew then they absolutely knew. But they decided to revive her anyway. Like, WTF?

When I walked into her room, her eyes literally lit up. Then she looked at me without a word and I saw her immense pain. I felt it hit my soul. The pain in her eyes told a story: *"I didn't want this. I didn't want to be here. And yet, here I am."*

I felt that everyone who knew her didn't respect her true feelings or beliefs beliefs she knew would end this way. For hours, I watched her try to be as happy as she could in the broken body she was trapped in. There was no saving her. My friend suffered eight long months of not being able to live, walk, smile, paint, or love deeply.

Jo was a very spiritual person right from the inner part of her soul. I'm not sure how to express the pain I felt during her last two weeks on earth. I may have mentioned it in an earlier chapter each time there was a new post, just an update but my heart sank every time I opened Facebook. The burden on my shoulders was heavy.

I felt her pain not being able to be *her*. I felt heartbroken because she couldn't paint, couldn't make music with her bowls, couldn't bring light to the world the way she always did. She brought so much light to everyone she met.

She loved with her whole heart through all her young years on earth. She never dwelled on the pain of the past. She simply put one foot in front of the other. She believed deeply in Mother Earth emotionally, physically, and spiritually. From the very day I met her, I was always in awe of her peaceful presence.

She is definitely at peace now, but she certainly left broken hearts behind. Our hearts will mend, and one day, we're told we will see them again.

I will take the best parts of knowing Jo and use that to heal my loss to heal the pain that only love can touch. Over the years, I've lost people family members, old school friends, and friends from our birthday group. There were ten of us who went to school together, all born the same day. It was truly fun back then.

As you navigate through life, remember it isn't always easy. Sometimes you have to fight. You have to stand up and use your backbone. You've made it just as far as I have. Don't let the bad energy in anymore. Let it go. You absolutely don't need it.

I got you. I'm proud of you proud of what you've walked through. Life will hand us some unmanageable moments, but that's when you grab hold of *you.* You are good enough. You are strong enough. You are certainly capable enough to take control of your life now.

Even when you're down reading my story, remember there will always be new days, new trauma, because that's just how the world is now. Hopefully, reading and listening to my voice as you go through these pages will give you some strength. Life is going to be hard, for sure. I can't stop bad things from happening death, heartbreak, broken promises but I can give you guidance.

We never need to bring our past back to life because it's already with us. It stays with us as long as we can remember those memories. No one can truly bring the past back, but we carry it within us. The past, the present, and the future they are separate, but they are all parts of us.

We never lose our past; it makes us who we are. We carry those memories forever.

The song *"Haunted by You"* sums up the love of your past, present, and future. Beautifully written it says it all if you really listen to the words and the voice singing them so eloquently.

Life will always hand you a few speed bumps along the way. Remember, they're only bumps in the road meant to make you slow down, focus, and breathe.

I will always have to work hard to move forward. I get up each and every day and give it my all, even with the heavy burden I still carry on my shoulders. Over time, yes, things do get lighter. You actually start to walk taller, shine brighter become that star you dreamed of being when you were young.

Over the years, I've seen, heard, and listened to endless stories of child abuse and neglect. I've watched one nationality receive national recognition and help for their suffering, and I've wondered: *What about everyone else?*

Even today, I ask myself why does only one group get support, compensation, and acknowledgment? Why not everyone who was damaged as a child? I don't sit here drunk or screaming about my terrible childhood. But why can one nationality be considered more important than another?

Why don't I get recognition for having my childhood stolen from me? Why is there someone remembered for every foot of the Canadian railway Chinese laborers who gave their lives for this country yet they were never recognized? Thousands of slaves lived and died before us in this country, and they weren't either. The injustice is astounding and no, not in a good way.

Why don't *we* ever get noticed? Why are so many people tossed aside like dirt on a shoe?

From where I stand and yes, I am educated on First Nations treaties and their history I can say that I have loved many friends from that culture. I even had an adopted sister who was Cree. I understand their pain. But I also feel the anger on both sides, because as we all grew, everyone absolutely 100% of the population had to learn that *many* suffered, *many* died, and *many* survived.

It's about time all the pain stops. We all chose, even through the treaties, to adapt and become part of society. The sad thing is hearing the stories where people still say, *"It's the white man's land."*

Life, married or not, is like a sailboat. Some days are smooth sailing, but then one day, a storm comes searching for attention, cutting off its anchor instead of adjusting its sails.

Sitting on the fence is okay. It gives you time to see what life is about to give you how life brings you forward to learn. Each moment of learning becomes a lifetime of meaningful memories. The moment you remember those lessons, you'll start to feel joy and happiness again.

Once you start to let go of what hurt you, love becomes easier. Love, in the end, is about forgiving it gives you the personal strength to move forward and live in the present.

You'll learn, just as I have well, shit, I'm still learning. When you stop learning, *then* be worried. Be present, and accept what's in front of you.

These days, I write because of the pain I carry. Writing has definitely been my process for handling my shit. *LOL.* It's been a good outlet a way to release, to let go, to finally put myself first.

Life will open doors for you when you're ready but remember, it will also close them. I've lived long enough to know that things happen for a reason. I truly believe, especially now, that in this day and age, we are all 100% responsible for our own actions.

Stop blaming everyone else for your choices and own them, as you should.

People and I mean *all* people need to own their shit. If someone caused your pain, then finally deal with it. You can't keep carrying it around forever. If you want to continue being angry, that's on you. If you cannot forgive again, that's also on you.

Reaching a milestone is an essential part of your freedom. Once you start doing the hard work, luck will begin to grow, and life won't feel as heavy or as hard as you think it is.

Maybe life *can* be different. Maybe life *can* change the direction in which you're headed. The path that brings you the most peace that's the one to follow.

Growing up is hard. Dealing with trauma is hard. But it's doable and it *can* be defeated.

As I'm writing all these pages, I've realized something important I haven't talked about survival with PTSD!

Chapter 10:
The Weight of Survival: A Lifetime of Trauma and PTSD

I think deep down, I've pushed this topic to the very bottom of my gut. From the depths of my soul, it breaks me to talk about that part of my life. Not only has it been heartbreaking, but it's also stolen the biggest part of me.

I've already suffered from depression all my life yeah, since I was seven way too young.

I've thought about exploring my life and pain through my writing. While I was writing, I started to talk about the depression part the hard part of living life but day by day, I kept pushing the *true* pain down deep. So deep that I learned to stay quiet.

But being silent nearly killed me. It gave me a stomach ulcer that almost took my life.

PTSD is absolutely a whole new universe a life-altering experience that you can't forget, no matter what you do. Before I was even old enough to start making good memories, those memories of growing up were stolen stolen by the very people who were supposed to love and protect us the most.

What the fuck did I do at eight years old to deserve being sexually abused? I was too young to have committed any kind of crime that would justify such inhumanity too young to lose who I was as a little girl.

I was robbed over and over again.

One day, a family was visiting, and we had a big canvas tent set up it could sleep ten people. I tried to run back to that tent, but I knew the heavy tree above it was about to fall. My Aunty Deb grabbed my hand and stopped me from running into what would have most definitely cost me my life. Sometimes, the cost of who you are can lead you toward a destination you never need to go.

Having to live through my devastating childhood losing my innocence before I was ready for the real pain that followed left scars too deep to fully explain. I can't put into words the kind of emotional and psychological pain I endured. I grew up under the false belief that *"things shouldn't be this way."*

Through my life growing, learning, and discovering pain I came to realize this:

Stop filling everyone else's cup. Let someone pour into yours.

Living with PTSD and depression is more than a daily challenge. Mine started when I was far too young much younger than anyone should ever have to experience. So early in life, my dreams turned into night terrors. By the time I was eleven, they came every night.

Oh, did it piss off my sister we shared a room. She lost a lot of sleepless nights because of me. My parents constantly yelled at me, telling me to *get over it.*

"Get over it?"

Fuck that.

The pain I endured year after year only added more fear. I learned to avoid sleep, because then I wouldn't have to wake up screaming, crying, and shaking uncontrollably. Every morning I woke up exhausted my body weak, my spirit tired. I was never without fear. I hadn't known love or peace only loss and anger.

When I woke up after falling off that cliff, I felt completely lost. I stood in the living room, scared and overwhelmed. My parents wouldn't listen to me. They just told me, again, *"Get over it."* For the first time, I had no idea what I was supposed to "get over."

That day, something inside me broke. I turned quiet. I turned inward. I became someone lonely and lost.

The years that followed passed slowly, filled with pain and suffering.

When I was sixteen, my health started to fail. I collapsed in gym class and was rushed by ambulance to a small clinic because the nearest hospital was already full of highway accident victims. The doctor asked me three simple questions, then told me I was bleeding internally from a stomach ulcer.

I was just twenty-one married for three years, with two kids under two when my husband began showing signs of emotional abuse. He called me unbelievable names, even in front of our children. Then one night, while I was sound asleep, he flipped my body over and started punching the shit out of me.

I finally got away, but he chased me through the house, catching me a few times each time, beating me worse. I spent that night huddled in a corner, waiting for the kids to wake up.

I can't count how many nights I woke up *feeling* like I'd been beaten again even when no one was there. If someone raised their hand near me, I'd flinch instantly. It took years to get over that kind of fear.

Years.

But from that day on, I made a promise to myself no one would ever raise their hands to me again.

As time passed, I learned to move forward to trust another man, slowly, after two long years of pain and healing. But even then, life

169

had more battles waiting. Within three years, I faced another: cancer.

It's hard enough to hear that word once but twice, in as many years? I was twenty-one, with an eighteen-month-old and a five-month-old. The diagnosis was breast cancer my left breast.

I was well-endowed, but I didn't care. I told the doctor immediately, *"Take whatever you need to and do it quickly."*

Within weeks, I had completed the mammogram and bloodwork to pinpoint the cancer. My ex-husband refused to take the kids, so I had to bring them with me. Talk about pressure two babies, and I had to fly to a major city for surgery.

My mother was still alive then. She helped me while I was in the hospital, but my emotions were all over the place. I didn't wake up easily from surgery and honestly, who would? Two kids under two I needed that nap. *LOL.*

Unfortunately, the people who were supposed to watch my back the ones only meant to give me the medicine I needed ended up nearly killing me. Some dumb fucken doctor gave me an overdose trying to wake me up. From that day forward, my body was never the same. It screwed me up in more ways than I can even write.

Now, I have deadly reactions to so many things. I have to carry an EpiPen at all times. What fun is that?

Because I was so broken on the inside and not mentally stable enough for another relationship, I made a mistake. I was drunk one night and ended up having a one-night stand that turned into a few more dates. Before I knew it, I was being told I was pregnant again.

No, it wasn't planned but I immediately accepted it.

Those months were brutal. I was emotionally abused almost daily, pregnant, and still raising two little ones. Every morning felt like climbing a mountain just to get out of bed. I tried so hard to find a way out, to move myself and my kids away from that abusive relationship.

Finally, with some help from my dickhead father, I managed to move. A few days later, I gave birth. My daughter came out blue, silent the room so still you could hear a pin drop. My heart sank deep into my stomach. Then, finally, she cried loud and strong and I broke down.

I was definitely suffering from postpartum depression, and on top of that, I was in terrible pain. My cervix felt like it was tearing apart. It hurt to sit, to walk, to pee everything hurt.

Living in a small town without an available OB-GYN made things worse. I had to drive to another town to get help. When I finally got a biopsy, the pain was unbearable worse than childbirth. The bleeding was so heavy that hospital pads couldn't even handle it. Days went by, and I lay in utter agony. They told me it would take four to six weeks to get results back.

That wasn't the case.

Five days later, I got a call telling me to come in immediately. My anxiety went through the roof. The 55-kilometer drive felt like forever. I sat in the office with a friend when the doctor came in, looked me dead in the eyes, and said,

"You have third-stage cervical cancer."

Then she added, "I won't do your surgery. I don't get paid for it."

Are you fucken kidding me? A doctor actually told me to find someone else.

Living far from any major city made finding another OB-GYN nearly impossible. I had three little kids, and chemo or radiation wasn't an option. I had no one the first time I fought cancer and no one the second time, either. I was beyond exhausted. Every day it got harder to keep going.

Then one afternoon, I made one last call and this beautiful soul answered. She listened as I told her everything. She put me on hold. I swear I was sweating bullets waiting for her to come back on the line. When she did, she said,

"When can you be here?"

I left the very next day a three-hour drive.

After I returned home, I had to take medication for thirty days that would make my body simulate a full-term pregnancy. They needed my belly expanded to make sure they could remove everything in one go. The surgery was supposed to take a few hours but ended up lasting seven.

When I woke up, the pain was unbearable. I screamed like never before. My lower back felt like it was on fire. They sent me for an X-ray and discovered I had an old fracture just above my tailbone.

I was surprised they released me the next day, but I could barely move because of the pain. My kids had a friend who agreed to help for a couple of days, but I ended up needing at least five. Recovery was brutal six long, painful weeks.

Then I got married again. We'd been together for two years before I said, *"I do."* I shit you not the day after, he flipped.

I didn't recognize the man I had married. Emotionally and physically, I spun out of control. He tore at my wellbeing, calling me names, breaking me down. One day he'd call me a slut, the next he'd demand I bring someone home for him to "watch." It was relentless pure emotional torture.

There were two times I gave in, completely broken, under duress. Weeks of abuse destroyed me from the inside out. My heart was shattered, my mind slipping, my body drained.

One day, I finally snapped. I sent my kids to a friend's house, gathered his things, threw them in the yard, and set them on fire. The only mistake I made was calling to tell him first so not much actually burned.

The next day was hot. I sat outside with my youngest, waiting for the older two to come home from school. My friend stopped by and asked if I needed anything. I said no.

Minutes later, I heard the sound of screeching tires an 18-wheeler trying to stop then the deafening crash of metal.

Then came the screams.

They cut through the air like nothing I'd ever heard. The neighbours were yelling, crying. The world went silent except for the sounds of snapping branches and the horrific wailing of a mother screaming, "No! No! No!"

I couldn't move. I dropped to my knees. I knew, without seeing it, that a mother had just lost her child.

That sound that cry still echoes in my dreams.

Even now, when I drive past that place, I can't help but think of that day. Think of that child. Think of the life that was lost and the mother who lost her will to live.

She was just a kid, riding her motorbike, when it stalled in front of an 18-wheeler.

My friend showed back up about half an hour later shaking, shivering, staring at his hands, crying uncontrollably. I reached out to hold him and asked if he was okay. That's when I saw the blood all over his hands, dripping down onto me.

My heart started racing a mile a minute. He collapsed into my arms, sobbing like I'd never heard before the kind of cry that comes from deep loss, fear, and absolute heartbreak.

After about ten minutes, he started to slow down, to breathe again. But as he pulled his hands toward him, the blood smeared down my arms, onto my back. He cupped his hands together and whispered, *"I held her. She was... crushed by the semi. Her brains were all over the road. I couldn't save her."*

Then the mother arrived barefoot, bleeding, her foot clearly broken. She tried to get to her daughter, but people wouldn't let her. I stayed with my friend. I called his wife, got him cleaned up before sending him home.

And yeah that night, we had a few beers and some really strong doobies. We needed it.

A couple of weeks went by before his wife called me again, terrified for his mental wellbeing. She said he couldn't stop seeing the scene couldn't stop smelling the blood. He was suicidal and needed help.

I spent the next three hours driving up and down dirt roads, trying to find the cliff where he was standing. There were a few cliffs where, if you jumped, you might never be found.

That night when I found him, he was almost beyond anyone's reach. His life meant absolutely nothing to him anymore not even his wife. The constant replaying of that moment, that smell of blood and iron... it haunted him. It made him sick, both mentally and physically.

The sadness we both felt that night was indescribable.

I had to keep it together. I had to remind him of the people who loved him, who needed him his wife, his family. What a battle it is, trying to hold someone back from jumping while you're also fighting your own darkness.

When you've shared a traumatic experience with someone, you understand the darkness they live in. You *feel* it with them.

In the weeks that followed, there were more nights where I had to go find him again and I always did. That accident changed us both. Forever.

To this day, it's hard to drive past that spot. I eventually moved away, but even now, whenever I have to pass through that town, the smell of iron fills my nose and the memories flood back.

My friend later asked me to come play a game of baseball they were short on players. So I said okay, packed up the kids, and went. My dad had taught me how to pitch, and I was damn good at it. Three up, three down no runs against us. We were kicking ass.

Then the coach from the other team told his batter to "hit the bitch."

The back catcher called us in and told us what the coach said. I couldn't believe it. *"No way,"* I said. *"He's standing there with a leg brace six feet tall! He wouldn't."*

My team begged me to sit down. I didn't. I didn't believe in my heart that anyone would actually do it.

I was wrong.

The first pitch he swung. The ball hit me dead on my left kneecap.

The impact lifted me right out of one shoe. I hit the ground hard, behind second base, and blacked out.

When I came to, the pain was indescribable the worst pain I'd ever felt. My leg was twisted, locked around the other. I tried to sit up, but all I could see was chaos everyone was fighting, yelling, swinging at each other. It was an all-out brawl.

I laid there crying, asking myself, *How could he? How could they play so dirty over a fucken baseball game?*

I had just healed after years of cancer and surgeries. Sports were my escape something I loved. And in a single moment, it was all taken from me.

That day changed my quality of life. It changed how I could play with my kids. I couldn't run, couldn't chase them around.

I fought the system for years to get my knee fixed. But every doctor kept saying the same thing *"You're too young. Take this pill, try that pill."* Always a no. Always a delay.

I didn't ask to be taken out like that. I didn't ask for a lifetime of pain at twenty-four.

By the time I was thirty-four, I was desperate begging for surgery, for a chance at a better life, for my kids' sake. Finally, after years of writing, screaming, crying, and begging, they said yes.

Yahoo!

But the joy was short-lived. The orthopedic surgeon I'd been seeing the one I trusted had his visa expire.

Who the fuck doesn't pay attention to those details?

My luck, right? So I get sent to a new doctor. He asks me a bunch of nonsense questions, then says, *"I won't do this surgery. You'll just need another one later in life. I can take a piece of your hip bone to buy you some time, but you'll end up with severe arthritis."*

I just sat there, numb.

For the second time in my life, the medical system told me *no.* The first time was cancer. This time, it was the chance to walk without pain.

Twice denied. Twice told my life didn't matter enough.

I was raising three kids, fighting depression, and recovering from cancer that had already taken everything even my ability to have more children. No one asked me if I was done having kids. They just took the choice away.

Life is never going to be easy not unless you were born with the right status. Life happens whether you want it to or not. It's always up to you to stand up, take a deep breath, and say, *"Fuck you. I'm done with your shit."*

Today is that day.

I am proud of you.

Life will challenge you to stand for who you are and face what comes your way. You got this.

I keep saying, *"You got this... I got you."*

Why? Because no one ever said it to me until one day, someone finally did. That changed everything. I've been writing every day since.

One day, you'll look at someone who's lost someone struggling to find themselves and you'll feel it in your heart to reach out. Use your voice, extend your hand, and just say, *"Hello."* That simple word might save their life.

One of the most intense traumas I've ever endured lasted for years. I would never wish it on another human being, no matter how inconsiderate they might be.

It started out as a normal, amazing day sitting around playing cards. My man's company called. After two quick questions, the line went dead. I jumped to my feet and started pacing the room, driving my roommate crazy with worry. I couldn't get through to anyone. Every number I tried was busy.

I sat down and smoked a joint to calm my nerves. The kids were getting ready for bed when the phone rang. It was the hospital the next town over, 55 kilometers away.

The nurse cleared her throat. She knew me her voice trembled.

"If you want to see him alive," she said quietly, "you need to get here immediately."

My heart dropped.

When I walked into the emergency department, the first thing I saw was blood. The floors were covered in it bloody footprints leading into a room. The trail of red told the story before anyone spoke.

A hand touched my shoulder as I looked through the doorway. My knees gave out. A nurse caught me before I hit the floor. But it was too late the image was already seared into my mind.

There were at least eight people working on him shouting orders, rushing around, covered in his blood. The smell hit me first thick, metallic, suffocating. My eyes burned from the sting of it.

I took a few steps forward, each one heavier than the last. His leg... it didn't even look like a leg anymore. The flesh was torn

178

open, blood spilling down the table drip, drip hitting the floor. I couldn't look away.

I forced myself to the side of the bed, leaned down, and whispered, *"It's okay. I'm here now. I got you. I love you."*

Then all the alarms started going off. Loud. Deafening.

He was in cardiac arrhythmia.

The team tried everything. Nothing was working. The doctor turned to me and said, *"Talk to him. Maybe your voice will calm him down."*

So I did.

And slowly finally his heart began to settle. The beeping slowed. His breathing steadied. After nearly two hours, he was stable enough to move.

As they wheeled him away, a nurse told me it would be a few hours before surgery was over. I went to the recovery floor to wait alone, falling apart.

Then another nurse walked down the hallway toward me, holding a yellow, see-through plastic bag. I could see the blood dripping inside. I could see bits of flesh.

Let me tell you if you ever have to deal with accidents like this, *don't look inside the bag.* Who the fuck cares what's in it? Your sanity isn't worth it.

But I did.

I opened it. I went through every bloody item pockets soaked in red, fabric stiff with blood. The smell hit me so hard I nearly vomited. That moment shattered something inside me. It was a sight you can't unsee a smell that never leaves you. Even now, the faintest trace of blood brings it all rushing back.

You'd think that was the end of it but no. It was only the beginning.

Every day, I drove between two towns 55 kilometers each way trying to balance the kids, the house, and my collapsing mental state. He'd been severely injured, and the local hospital wasn't equipped to handle it.

The arrogance of some of the staff was unreal. One doctor even said to my face, *"If this were me, I'd ask to be transferred to a bigger city."*

I couldn't believe what I was hearing. They admitted they couldn't handle it yet still refused to move him.

For three weeks, I lived through hell, trying to get him transferred. Something in me that gut instinct told me to take pictures. So I did.

When I finally broke down completely, I went to WorkSafeBC with the photos. I had a full-blown nervous breakdown right there in their lobby sobbing, screaming, shaking. People came running.

Within an hour, there was a bed waiting for him in the city.

They arranged the airlift, and I was sent on a regular flight. It took me six long, painful hours to reach his bedside.

When I got there, they had placed him in the burn unit the smell of his wound was unbearable. The first surgeon had stitched him up without removing the dead tissue. Three weeks later, that tissue was rotting. The damage was catastrophic.

Every time I entered the room, I had to gown up completely gloves, mask, the works. I had to be buzzed into the ward just to see him.

It was extremely hard every single day going through the process of watching him suffer in so much pain. The doctors had him on a pain-release system where he could press a button to give himself medication. That medication was heroin.

After weeks of using it, he started having night terrors, sweating through the sheets, and living in a constant fog.

Sitting by his bedside day in and day out was emotionally exhausting. The overwhelming feeling of helplessness not being able to ease his pain was unbearable.

Every day was filled with more appointments, more tests, more procedures, as doctors tried to figure out the best plan to help him heal. We spent the next three weeks going back and forth between treatments and evaluations.

Finally, it was time to go home but with conditions.

I had to give him his medication directly into his stomach every six hours. I had to change his bandages from the knee down, and I also had to administer saline when he was weak.

We hadn't even been home for three days before he started having full-blown seizures. He had never had them before.

I tried to help him, but the kids heard him fall and came running. They started screaming the whole house turned to chaos. I was on the phone with the ambulance, trying to calm them while making sure he didn't swallow his tongue.

Experiencing seizures for the first time I was losing my grip, losing my sanity. I felt like I had no control over our lives anymore.

Every time I had to call an ambulance, my heart broke a little more. I would explain how big he was he wasn't some 165-pound man but they'd still send one small woman or a smaller man to lift him. It was torture watching him suffer and having to wait twenty minutes for more help, even though the hospital was just a block away.

His leg was never amputated because, unbelievably, the bone didn't break.

How did it happen?

He worked at a well-known aluminum plant. His leg was crushed between his step and the bumper of another vehicle. The truck's reverse alarm the *beep beep* didn't work. They stopped the truck by jumping on the hood, but in his shock, he stepped forward and *boom*. His leg was impaled into his work pants, and he collapsed.

Even today, he still struggles walking, sleeping, dealing with swelling, shadow pain, drop foot. He lost so much that day because of someone else's negligence.

The trauma also hit the kids hard. Every time he had a seizure, every hospital visit, every late-night emergency it broke them a little more too.

The years that followed were brutal. They stretched me further than I ever thought possible.

I was raising kids, working, and going back to school. One day, I stopped just outside the school doors. It was snowing hard, the wind howling, and I just collapsed into the snow emotionally drained. I started crying, screaming, shaking. I had reached my breaking point the end of my patience. I dug deep inside myself to try one more time to keep going.

After everything that had happened with his accident, I found out he'd started using cocaine without me knowing.

I realized it when I reached into my pocket to grab the money I needed to pay the mortgage… and it was gone.

I was beyond angry. I was beyond caring about how he was doing. I was consumed by rage pure, uncontrollable anger.

A few days later, on New Year's Day, there was loud banging at my side door.

When I opened it, there stood a police officer and another woman holding a big black binder. My anxiety went through the roof.

They said, "We need to speak to you about a few incidents in the house."

Are you fucking kidding me?

They proceeded to tell me that my son and foster son had taken advantage of my stepdaughter.

Can you imagine?

Fire ripped through my body. I couldn't breathe. There was *no fucking way in hell.*

I had been raped. I knew that kind of pain. I never wanted to be in the same room let alone live in the same house with anyone who could do that to another person.

I put all the cards on the table and demanded answers. Both boys had to go through hours of questioning. I called her mother and told her, *"You better be here in ten minutes, because I'm about to beat the fuck out of her."*

That fuck face ran straight out the door.

It took me over ten years to speak to her again. And even now, she's fake as hell. She plays the depressed card, uses everyone around her, manipulates, lies and I will never trust her again.

She will never have my respect. I will never help her in any way. Selfish individual.

Because of her actions and her father's I decided that day to end things.

It was New Year's Day.

Then, as if on cue, he dropped to the floor another full seizure. Teenagers were yelling, crying, fighting. I called an ambulance again and told one of the kids to call their dad.

At the hospital, his father showed up. He looked at me and said, "What's wrong? You don't look good either."

I fell to my knees, crying. *"I'm broken,"* I said. *"I can't hide anymore. I can't keep this from you."*

He sat down beside me. I wiped my tears and told him everything what the police had said about his grandchild, and about his son's addiction to cocaine.

He hung his head. I had never seen disappointment like that in anyone's eyes before.

I took a deep breath, hugged him, and said, *"When he gets out of the hospital, I won't be home. I'm moving out."*

I walked away from everything. I left the house with all the belongings and started over again. My girls were so disappointed with me and didn't understand why. So for weeks they cursed me out and totally pushed my buttons to piss me off. My youngest thought she would set me up to find her losing her virginity. Right, fuck me. I picked that boy up and threw his ass down those stairs.

I had moved to the island and my girls came soon after. So we moved into a bigger house and one day my girls were sitting in the garage smoking and toking. I decided to join them for a smoke and my youngest did this bong hit, but it didn't smell like weed. I asked what it was and apparently it was legal and sold in head shops. They told me to try it at a different height. It lasts like thirty seconds.

It was thirty seconds I can never go back. I can never undo that torturous, life-shattering moment for me. I literally have to stop and smoke a joint to relive this part! I took a toke from the bong. In my mind I believed it would be just like a quick hit of pot.....I was suddenly burning in the core of my body. I started sweating; I was burning up. I kept pushing back as I was stripping because of my inner heat.

All I felt from my inner body was total and utter fear. Flashing right in my face was all my younger years: the sexual abuse I pushed deep down, the constant raping I endured before the age of twelve. The moment I realized I was never loved as a child was the loneliness, the utter feeling of betrayal from all my family. All the beatings I endured. Tremendous pain was rushing through me; it was rushing through my veins.

I was completely outside by the time I regained consciousness from that terrible experience. I only had my shirt on, standing in the rain looking at my kids about forty feet from me. I pushed myself that far during that simple thirty-second high that literally sent me in a spiral. I was so overwhelmed I left them instantly. I was literally in an emotional breakdown. Every single event in my life before I was twelve was visually devastating. I couldn't talk; breathing was so hard, just gasping for a breath.

I went to my room and I shut the door. I crawled under my blanket. I thought if I just went to sleep this would just be a nightmare. Not so lucky…I was up and down every half hour, waking up in fear, waking up sweating like no tomorrow. I was soaked; I was scared; I was deeply broken all over again. I had a week of not getting up, not doing anything; my state of mind emotionally was exhausted.

I didn't know what was true and what was not. All I knew deep within me is that was my childhood; I wasn't someone I loved; I wasn't protected. I remembered the fall of the cliff and how much it hurt hitting the cement cylinder, blackberry bushes, and tons of discarded material. I remembered even who carried me home. I realized that's why I never remembered my early years.

For years I wondered why I was a little colder than most people. I finally got my answer. Not only did I get raped when I was a teen, but then I remembered how young it started. I was sick; I was in a state of breaking my soul, to have it in front of my face as it was happening now….watching almost in real time when the abuse started, then the raping started.

I was fucken only a kid; I wasn't even eight; I wasn't even old enough to kiss, yet the people close to me and my sister decided to use us as guinea pigs to learn…The anger grew fast, uncontrollable. I kept having an anxiety attack reliving every time I closed my eyes. I was trying to be in denial, so I called my sister who was with me when we first started getting abused. She calmly said yes!

I couldn't swallow; I couldn't breathe; it felt like my heart dropped to my toes. I fell to the ground and I asked, "Why did you not say anything?" She said, "I didn't know how. I wasn't sure what was happening." My heart was racing so fast; my anxiety was way out of control. I was screaming deep inside my heart, knowing no one stood up for us. No one protected us. No one loved me enough.

I was already suffering from a depressive state as I left my third husband shortly before this. My heart was far beyond mending; the heartbreak tore my life apart. The visions in my head were very vivid; daily and weekly they consumed my every moment. I was in a daily tornado in my life; at this point, finding peace, finding closure just wasn't in the cards I knew it then. I knew deep down at some point in my life I need to let it go. Because it's family, I do not know if I can break my father's heart. To know two of his nephews abused his girls; they took the innocent; they robbed us of purity.

I completely lost myself all over again; it felt like someone reached into my chest and yanked my beating heart out. Any chance I had when no one was around, I would go into my room, cover my face with my pillow, and cry. It definitely took some time to come out of that emotional pain. My heart sank; my pain, my soul was shattered; I wasn't sure I would recover. Parts of me will always be working on healing.

The most pain I felt was the deepest part of who I had become. A Nana is a completely devoted one. I changed my life to become his permanent caregiver. My wellbeing needed him, my precious grandson. In my heart was learning to forgive; it was learning unconditional love all the way. I was being robbed of who I was trying so hard to be because my fucken daughter decided to have an affair and made me keep quiet.

My anger started to build up, day after day of being asked to lie… I left lying behind decades ago; it served no purpose but more heartbreak. My internal struggles were hard to handle. Christmas was coming and my son-in-law's mother was coming. Oh fuck, she was definitely a hard one to deal with.

I was so broken that morning, again another year of me doing everything for this child, for her children, all child care. I went above and beyond at Christmas and my selfish daughter gave me literally gifts from the fucken dollar store. WTF, again!!! I was so angry. No, it wasn't about the gift; it was the lack of love, appreciation, just a little. It was the same every year. I felt used, I felt unloved and unappreciated.

I got up, went for a smoke; I had to breathe. It felt like I was drowning; I was drowning in the constant feeling of not being loved. My grandson walked out to the patio and came up and kissed me. It instantly calmed me down. Suddenly everyone was outside having a smoke and I simply said, "You best tell him or I will." That fucken kid even made me say it… that she was sleeping around!

Within seconds my life was never the same. I was kicked out of the house and told to leave while my grandson was sitting on me, hugging me, telling me he loved me. Oh, my heart broke; I fell to the ground gasping for air; I literally couldn't breathe. Watching my son-in-law hold him back from giving me one last hug, one last moment.

For three days I lived on the streets. Oh, my fear, my heart was shattered; my train of thought wasn't even processing anything. I cried for days until one day I couldn't help it, but my fear of my mental wellbeing had no concept of knowing I could get through it. I set everything up just to end things as easily as it was, meaning I could get rid of the pain.

I had already lost my other granddaughter because of my narcissistic kid. She is a completely different story on a whole new level. I haven't spoken to her in nine years. No, I do not miss her; I miss my grandchild though. I miss the time we could have made amazing memories. Those will have to wait for another day.

I know I didn't give my kids the easiest life, but I tried, and the one thing I absolutely did not do was use the kids as pawns. My girls used their children just like that. They both need to be slapped, and honestly, the judge in any case with my grandkids needs to be absolutely fucken fired. Shame on you all!

The true emotional, physical, and mental abuse my girls have done to me has broken me to the very centre of my being. These two, true narcissists all the way. My older daughter disgraced her man. My son-in-law was definitely an amazing father who was dragged through the mud over lies, the grandkids suffering at their mother's hands, not just with the change in relationship with their dad but also with their Nana.

If the Nana was always the babysitter, I did the pick up, sleepovers, I did everything as a Nana should. Then, all because I corrected the kids on a visit, the kids stated that their mom couldn't use the EpiPen? Confused, I asked why? They explained to me that their mother said she is allergic to it. Holy fuck! I told the kids their mother is misinformed. I stated no one on earth is allergic whatsoever to an EpiPen.

I have never seen my grandkids since; not a call was returned from my kid. She blocked me on all social media. She absolutely took the cunt way; she hurt me in the inner core with the kids. My heart aches for the two birthdays I have missed with my grandson. I cannot explain the relationship I have with my grandson. The pain causes my depression to flare. The bad memories of loss running through my mind; the pain running through the deepest parts of my heart.

The parents that use children as the tool should be the ones who lose custody, absolutely no question asked. Why do I say that? Because doing so only leads to mind games and completely bullshit from the ex. Seriously, if you are going against a total bitch, please use all your strength to take her down. We know she's fucken lying. Being lied to over and over again and changing the way people see you is extremely hard to take control of.

The system has failed more men than I can count and has shelved more grandparents even further away. Judges for sure have a grueling job, but you have neglected the most important aspect of the   children.
Yes, I am still angry; I have tried a thousand ways to get over it and I cannot. Depression has taken hold of me and I truly do not know how to let this emotional state go.

I have to stop writing. My heart is hurting; my eyes are filled with tears I cannot stop. The true emotional heartache of not seeing them, them not seeing me. My daughter is not giving a true reason other than her fucken bullshit lies. The anger mixed with my heartbreak over true pain consumes me. I cry myself to sleep almost every night.

I suppose my heart breaks more because my grandkids' pictures fill my place. They are my picture home page. My peace and my external happiness is with the grandkids. I was motivated to get up every single day, but not over the last year. My faith, my dreams, wishes, and all the begging has led to no chance of seeing the most special people in my life. They were my reason for living.

I get up without a purpose; I get up without the feeling of being loved, no inner purpose to move forward each day. I felt lost, defeated; each day my heart breaks. My reason to move forward is not on my path so much.

Getting up literally every day knowing I'm missing people who truly love you unconditionally. I have lost. I need that back; I need that love; they know I am there for them. The feeling of loss between their father and me. Oh fuck, that kid, I seriously could beat her. Leaving that relationship was the hardest one out of all my so-called marriages. I truly loved him, but he broke my spirit. I had to move forward in order for my mental wellbeing.

By this time I was so emotional and physically drained, I was helpless. I was not really connected to myself; my depression, my anxiety, my fears were all in full force of taking control of my entire existence. It took me a few years to get back on my feet. It took time for me to let go of the anger, the disappointment, the heartbreak.

For the third time I walked away with only my children's belongings. All the rest are the material things I left behind. Sometimes life is just hard, even harder for others. The constant search through my life searching for the simplest thing…..love! I still haven't found it. Sometimes I think I missed that part in my life since the very day I was born. Maybe it just isn't in the cards for me. Maybe I have just always had the wrong idea on what love should be, how it should feel.

A few years passed and I did the stupid thing and got married again. I always believed that I would only be happy while I was married. I received a call from my grandmother asking for help. She would never ask, let alone me, the black sheep. But I drove eight hours and got to my grandmother's. She filled me in on my mother, the one I hadn't spoken to in over ten years.

My grandma was at her wit's end, so I went to the hospital where she is, and I could hear her screaming from the entrance of the hospital. I walked into her cubicle and she literally says, "Why the fuck are you here?" I took a breath and said I would go get her something, so I bought her her favourite chocolate bar. I got back to her space and she was still arguing with the doctors, and he threw his hands up and walked away.

I gave my mom the chocolate bar and she started on me, telling me how much of a disappointment I was and how she has regretted my existence. I got up and started to walk away and this four-foot-eight little old lady with no teeth started chasing me down the hall, throwing things at me, yelling how much she hated me, how much she wished I would just go.

Security came and he stopped me and asked if I was okay? He said he has never witnessed something so horrible to another person. He had tears in his eyes looking at my pain. She just kept yelling everything she could think of. For the next five days it would just repeat like the first. My mother was on a mission to take her life and so yelled loudly every day, but no, they wouldn't put her in a psych ward because she refused.

My mom got me good. In the end she called the cops on my grandma, who sold a bit of pot. Oh, my grandma was furious with me. She 100% blamed me, like WTF, I was a pot smoker, why the fuck would I? But she never believed me and she was never the same with me. Well, we never had much of a relationship because of my mother and, well, shit I pulled when I was a child!

I cannot explain the pain I felt every time my family got together. I watched everyone be loved, hugged, smothered with affection right in front of me. I never got held or loved like that. That inner hurt of anger really doesn't ever go away.

A few years later my grandmother had a brain aneurysm. My sister and I went to the hospital; as the day passed more family showed up, each one giving my sister hugs and affection, while I stood against the window. One by one we said our goodbyes. As I said mine I told my Gran why I did the first thing I ever did, and that was steal 50 from my cousins in her home. My Gran had tears running down her face.

I was taken back; I realized that she could hear us. As we all gathered back into her room, my aunts, cousins, uncles, except for one, were all hugging and kissing. One of my uncles finally lost it...I never thought I would ever see the day someone would stick up for me. He yelled, "She is here too, you all should be ashamed." I had to leave the room. That night our Granny passed.

The next day we all met at another aunt's house. Why did I even think things would be different, but nope…everyone hugging, kissing, reminiscing together. I was once again pushed into a corner. After a few hours I couldn't do it anymore: the coldness, the lack of empathy, the total disbelief that even in the eyes of death I will always be alone. We had my daughter's car so my sister needed to drive me back home.

That was an hour-and-a-half trip where I seriously considered jumping out of the moving car. My sister attacked me. She yelled and yelled at me how worthless I was and how much the family dislikes me. "Not a single soul trusts you; they don't like being around you; they believe you will never change. Why did you even bother coming when no one wanted you here, couldn't you tell?" Believe me, more was said, but trying to write that I cannot stop crying. To this very day my mind can hear every word and can remember every single stab in my heart.

When I got home, my daughter could tell something was seriously wrong with me. I went straight to my room, shut the door, and cried all night. The next day, I couldn't get out of bed. My body was mentally exhausted, and I was in physical pain. My heart had never felt such enormous hurt.

A few weeks later, they held the celebration of life at my uncle's place. First, there was the memorial service at the funeral home. My family filled the first two rows, all nestled together. As I walked past one of my aunts, she actually turned her face away.

After the service, everyone was supposed to meet at my uncle's house. But as I was leaving, my mother started yelling at me across the parking lot, filled with family and friends. Her voice carried that deep, hateful tone that pierced right through me. As she walked closer, the yelling grew louder. Everyone turned to look at me standing there, holding my grandson.

I told my daughter, *"It's time to go."*

It was the first time my mom had seen her granddaughter in over ten years, and it would have been the very first time she met her great-grandson but fuck no, she ruined it.

I can't count how many times I've had to stop writing just to catch my breath and wipe away tears. The pain of loss still finds its way to the surface. Getting over things, holding on to hope it always takes time. There's no cure for this kind of pain. Remember that.

You just have to keep finding ways to put one foot in front of the other. There's a reason you're here. There's a purpose for you for all of us. You still need to find that, just as I'm still trying to find mine.

It's going to be fucking hard some days, but some days will also be amazing.

One day, out of the blue, I got a call from my aunt the same aunt who had *never* called me before. She was my godmother, yet she'd turned her back on me when I was thirteen. She told me my mother was dying and said I'd better be ready to go to Kamloops the next morning. Her voice was stern, cold.

My anxiety kicked in instantly. My chest was tight, my heart was pounding, and I started sweating. I couldn't imagine spending six hours trapped in a truck with two aunts who made me feel like I had nowhere to run.

My emotions were spiraling. I was on my way to see a mother I hadn't seen in years who was now dying and I had to do it surrounded by people who never liked me.

During the drive, my sister told me something I'd never known. She said my aunt had hated me since I was thirteen because she thought I'd stolen her jeans. I hadn't. I was barely a hundred pounds there was no way I could have fit into her jeans. But she never said a single word to me about it. She just cut me off all those years ago.

Sitting behind her in that truck, I was breaking down inside.

Every second I spent in that house, I felt unwanted. I felt completely out of place.

The next day, we went to the hospital to see my mom. She was so tiny maybe seventy-five pounds, frail and fragile, trying to hold her oxygen mask in her hand. It was a child-sized mask, small and out of place on her face. For a split second, I thought she smiled at me, but her brother was standing beside me, so maybe she didn't.

For a couple of days, it looked like she might improve, but it didn't last. We called the priest to give her last rites. All five of us kids stood around her bedside while her brother and sisters stood at her feet.

The nurse came in, unplugged the machines, and gently took the oxygen from her hands. It only took a few moments. Her lungs just stopped. No deep breath, no sound just silence.

I was overwhelmed being there after she passed. The very next day, I had to help clean out her apartment so they could rent it again. The pressure was crushing. But at least the family did a small honoring for her. My brother poured us each a shot, said a few words, and that was it.

After that, I only went to one family gathering. You'd think I'd have learned my lesson by then, right? But my daughter wanted to go.

My aunt the same one who could never let go of anything was there too. Funny how she could forgive everyone else's mistakes but never mine. I was just a kid.

I went straight to the farthest picnic table and sat down. I watched everyone hugging, laughing, loving each other. No one came to me until my only uncle, the one who truly loved me, showed up. For a fleeting moment, I felt what love was again.

As I sat there, my cousin approached me and asked softly, *"Can we talk?"*

No cousin had ever asked to talk to me before maybe once or twice in my life, but never like this. I was hesitant, unsure of her reason, until she looked at me and asked, *"How have you handled being the black sheep all these years? Does it ever change? Does the family ever forgive and forget?"*

Her eyes filled with tears, her voice trembling as she tried not to cry. She quickly turned away and wiped her face.

My heart sank. It was beating so fast I could barely think. Finding the right words wasn't easy. But I knew I had to tell her the truth to give her something to hold on to, even if I couldn't fix her pain.

I told her what I'd learned: that sometimes people can change, but often, it just takes time and forgiveness, even when it's hard.

She shared her story with me her battles, her addiction, her pain. And my heart broke into a million pieces as I listened. I could see the same kind of hurt I'd carried for years reflected in her eyes.

She cried and said, *"My God, I can't believe this is how you felt all your life."* Then she wrapped her arms around me and whispered, *"I'm sorry."*

I couldn't fix her pain. I didn't have the answers oh, how I wish I had. But I told her one thing I truly believed: *"Don't give up. People just need time to let go."*

I truly believed she would be forgiven that she was still very much loved by the whole family. I mean, we were at her birthday party too.

A few weeks later, my brother called me to tell me our cousin had overdosed. She was in the hospital on life support. A few days later, she passed. She was truly a beautiful soul.

That was the last family gathering I went to thirteen years ago now.

No, I don't miss it. I don't miss the enormous pain I always felt when I was around them. I don't miss watching everyone else be loved while I stood there invisible. I no longer have to feel them walk right past me like I'm some fucking ghost.

When my favorite aunt passed away, not one person called, texted, or even emailed me. My other aunt the same one who'd turned her back on me told me *on Facebook.*

The pain cut deep, like being stabbed in the heart with a jagged knife.

I remember sitting down when I read the news. My heart sank, and I began to cry uncontrollably for a long time. She only lived less than an hour away from me.

I keep asking myself, *Have you forgiven? Have you really let go?* Some days I think I have, and then I drive past her home, and the ache comes rushing back.

The grief of not being able to say goodbye never goes away. I never got to tell her that she was my favorite person. I was robbed of that chance robbed of saying goodbye, robbed of saying thank you for loving me when no one else did.

I didn't get one last hug. Not one last kiss.

I've always felt like I missed an important moment one that I need to finally lay to rest. I've accepted the lack of empathy from my family. It's been a long road, but I've stopped expecting it.

This past year has been extremely difficult emotionally and physically. My wellbeing was shattered when my daughter, once again, took the kids away. It's been devastating.

I was a hands-on Nana. The loss of their unconditional love broke my heart. Not being able to watch them grow, to see their milestones, has been soul-crushing.

My daughter used my love for those kids as a weapon to hurt me, and in doing so, she hurt them too. The things she did were malicious. She caused extreme anxiety and depression in her own children. It breaks my heart every minute of every day. Keeping children away from family from the love and support they need is something no one should ever do.

Over this last year, my self-esteem, my confidence, and my sense of self-worth have all taken major hits.

In the span of just two weeks, I lost two amazing people. Both of them loved with complete, unconditional hearts.

I've fought many battles some I wasn't sure I'd survive. Battling depression on top of PTSD has been crippling. There were times I didn't think I could go on. My anxiety has been so extreme that I didn't know how to handle it emotionally.

There were moments I thought, *maybe my pain would finally stop if I wasn't here anymore.*

198

But even through that darkness, I knew there were still three people who truly loved me my grandkids and my son.

They're my reason.

My mental health has been fighting me every day this past month, but I keep trying.

Throughout the decades of my life, I've been challenged from the very beginning. My earliest memories are filled with disappointment. I was no longer "Daddy's little girl." That love was short-lived.

No one was ever there to protect me.

From childhood to adulthood, my life has been harder than I could have ever imagined. The constant pain has shaped me into a strong but broken woman one who never truly had a chance to begin with.

For many, many years, I've suffered from night terrors waking up drenched in sweat, my body cold, my mind trapped in confusion, trying to escape memories that won't stay buried. Those memories turn into nightmares, and those nightmares drain the life out of you.

I try every day to move forward. Some days I do. Some days, I don't move at all.

Depression is the biggest hurdle you'll ever face.

Depression and PTSD together can tear you apart emotionally, mentally, and physically. They drain your spirit. They steal your focus. They paralyze your will to keep going. Anxiety takes control, blocking your power to move forward. It stops you from taking that next step.

Some days, you will fall. And that's okay. Let yourself feel it. Then, when you can, let it go.

Can I tell you it's going to be easy? No. I can't even imagine what *you* might be going through. But we each have our own story to tell.

Each of us is at a different stage in life. I've been through horrific, cruel things. I was stripped of my innocence before I even had the chance to say no. But I survived.

It took me a long time to understand that you don't necessarily need your family.

Sometimes, you'll realize that you can't keep being around the people who hurt you. You only get one life. Live it for *you.*

Not for the people who talk behind your back. Not for the ones who always let you down.

Only *you* can change your story. Only *you* can rewrite the path you're on.

Being true to yourself has to come first even if it means losing loved ones along the way.

If they won't stand beside you, reaching out their hand to help you grow, then let them go.

If you've noticed the people you keep giving to over and over again   ask   yourself   this: **What have they ever done for you?**

Have they extended their hand when you needed them?

Have they shown up when you were falling apart?

Probably not.

There will always be times when you hear something on the news, or see posts on Facebook, TikTok, or anywhere else that make you stop and think.

If life were meant to always be easy, then we'd never learn a damn thing. Lessons are what shape us. You're not the only one suffering or struggling there are so many others, we've just all had different journeys. Some lessons are hard to learn, but finding peace within that pain *that's* when you start to heal.

As the years have gone by, I've seen things that shocked me to my core. People I thought were untouchable people who seemed so full of life were battling the same darkness I knew all too well.

Robin Williams was the biggest shock to me.

When I heard that depression had taken him, my heart broke. I felt that pain deep in my soul.

Patience. Loyalty. Trust. Love.

Those things aren't always unconditional.

If people don't have those qualities when it comes to *you*, then there's no reason to keep them in your life. If they haven't stood by your side by now, chances are they never will.

It's up to you who you let in.

There will be people who stand beside you, and there will be people who secretly want to see you fail.

Sometimes life is going to be *hard*. It's going to feel like nothing is going your way. Stop. Take a breath.

How you move forward from that moment will define who you become in the end.

It's time to take control even when it's hard. Get up. Deal with it. Find a way to let it go.

Sometimes it'll take you two tries. Sometimes three. But as long as you *keep trying*, that's what will change your future.

Life will change.

Life will change *you*.

And when it does, that's your cue to trace a new path or cut away what's been weighing you down. Some choices won't be easy. Some will test your peace. Some will almost break you.

But you have control.

You have more control now because you know *you're not alone.*

Living with depression or PTSD doesn't define who you are meant to be.

You are your own guiding light.

Believe in yourself. Believe that you deserve better. Believe that you deserve unconditional love.

Travelling through my life, I've learned many hard lessons and made some amazing memories too.

Sometimes it's hard to remember who I wanted to be when I grew up. But one thing I can say for certain I didn't want to be an anxiety-ridden, sarcastic, tired-as-hell woman who's had to claw her way through everything.

Through it all, I've learned how to tell people to fuck off without ever having to say a single word.

It's better to tell the truth than to bite my tongue, because honestly?

It bleeds way too much.

I no longer have the energy to keep pointing out what people do wrong.

It's painfully exhausting.

Chapter 11:
The Reckoning: Forging a New Self from the Broken Pieces

Every story is different.

In many situations, the emotional part is draining it consumes you.

Remember this: **a mistake made more than once is no longer a mistake it's a decision.**

Repeat it three times, and it becomes a habit.

Keep going, and it starts to build your character.

If I had never experienced being broken, I would never have known how to heal. If I had never been lost, I would never have understood what it truly means to hold on.

This new version of me has inspired me.

My story, I hope, reaches many people. There was once a version of me who didn't know how to stand on her own. Now, I hope others can see strength in my words.

There are still nights when I sit in silence alone with the wisdom I've gained along my journey. I just hope you don't hear the echoes of everything I once questioned.

Through all my lessons, I've realized one of the best things I've learned is simply this: **enjoy life**, even in the middle of your storms.

Our problems don't always go away, but even when your world feels chaotic, you can still find moments to laugh, moments to smile.

Even on the hardest days, I've learned that I prefer a quiet life.

I stopped chasing friendships and relationships.

Having fewer friends made me happier.

Leave the drama behind.

Be the best version of yourself.

Stop comparing your life to others and start enjoying your own company.

You can make yourself happier than anyone else ever could.

One of my biggest regrets will always be that I didn't know how to value myself that I didn't realize my worth was so much more than what I was given.

I hope you don't have to learn the way I did through loss, heartbreak, and pain.

Let me be the first to tell you, if no one ever has:

You are worthy.

You are valued.

You are everything you need to be.

If you're unsure which road you're walking, pursue *you.*

Pursue yourself now, in the present.

Learn to love yourself.

Become the confident version of who you were meant to be.

The right path will appear when you finally do.

One day, you'll look back for that old version of yourself the broken, lost, lonely one and you'll realize they're gone.

All that's left is the stronger, wiser, better version of you.

Now you're standing on your own. You feel whole again.

You're healing in the best way you know how.

The old you taught you enough to survive the storm.

The new you?

She's here to *live* through the calm.

She'll bring laughter, light, and far less pain to carry.

Most importantly, she'll bring you peace.

As the old saying goes:

Everything happens for a reason.

That includes the highs, the lows, the wins, and even the losses including the people you've had to let go because of their drama.

Nothing in life is random. Every moment good or bad carries a lesson. Each lesson will guide you, hold your hand, and help you find your true purpose.

When life gets heavy, stop. Pause. Breathe.

There's always a lesson waiting inside the weight.

At some point, you need to forgive yourself for all your past mistakes.
Release the anxiety that's been building up inside you.

Start focusing on *now.*

Right here, right now this is what truly matters.

If you keep falling back into the past, or racing ahead into the future, you'll waste your energy and your peace.

And the only thing you'll lose is **today's calm.**

Start living *today.*

Be the reckoning they'll never forget.

Be the person who finally rewrites their world.

One day, you'll wake up and realize you're in the right place that everything around you finally feels right.

The new you will have a calmer heart, positive thoughts, and a vision that finally came to life.

It took me years to get here, all on my own.

But I am so grateful I did.

I know there will always be people who think my life will never get better but it will.

Let me be that voice on your shoulder.

Let me walk with you toward your peace toward the freedom that comes when you finally put down your burdens.

After everything you've been through, seen, and felt let it fade into the past.

Accept that not all days will be good days. We fall as we grow. But if we learn, if we heal, we'll fall less over time.

Mistakes happen.

We fail.

We mess up.

It's okay.

Because that's how we learn.

Finding truly loyal friends is hard.

I've learned that the people who call themselves friends aren't always the ones who care. I found out the hard way what a *real friend* means.

Oh boy, did I ever get fucked over.

But now, I know better.

I know what to look for.

A real friend is someone who takes ownership of their actions who's accountable, honest, and genuine. Someone who *shows up.*

Find the people who match their words with their actions.

Find the ones who care about what's happening in your life, who listen, who understand.

Growing up, I was taught that if I treated people with kindness, they'd return it.

Boy, was that a letdown.

Life showed me otherwise.

People are people some act with heart, others act only for themselves. They don't care how their behavior affects others.

But at the end of the day, **actions speak louder than words.**

And those who speak the loudest negativity? Their words mean the least.

I never knew what it felt like to be valued but I learned.

I learned that the people who value your time, your presence, and your energy are the ones who truly matter. No matter what's going on in life, always choose to be *valued.*

My story has been about healing, finding myself, learning to finally love myself, and choosing *me* without apologizing for who I am.

If you've made it this far, then you must want to know you want to hear what life is really here to give you.

You're ready now.

Start today. Let go of one thing.

Let today be the beginning of your new story the story of finding yourself, loving yourself, and being at peace.

You can be whoever you want to be beautiful, happy, worthy, a total kick-ass individual.

If only we could skip the hardest pages of our story... but we can't.

We have to keep moving one foot in front of the other.

Like me, you might not love every part of your journey. Some parts will hurt. Some will make you cry. Some will make you want to give up.

But in the middle of those hard days, you'll find small moments that turn into beautiful memories moments you'll wish would never end.

That's why you have to keep going.

Some people today don't even realize what *survival* looks like. Some will still judge you without ever walking a single day in your shoes. They have no idea what struggling means or what being broken really feels like.

There will always be people who want to see you fall.

I've felt alone, even when surrounded by friends. But after getting back up again and again, I've learned something important:

Every time you fall, rise again.

And each time you rise, rise higher than before.

Rise and show your beauty. Show your strength.

Never care about the ones who leave the loyal ones will stay.

They've seen you at your worst, yet they still see the beauty in you that others can't.

When I meet new people who want to be friends, I tell them the truth *I don't let many people into my circle.*

Now that I know better, I've learned the lesson of friendship the hard way.

I'll be honest I've said things I didn't mean. I've lost control when my emotions got the best of me. My personality changes with my mood.

I've been mean. I've made grown men cry.

My words can cut deep when I'm hurt or cornered. I know how dangerous my tongue can be.

That's why I've learned to stay quiet sometimes.

Because words can wound deeper than any weapon.

We all need to think before we speak to focus more on *how* we say things than on the anger we want to show.

Time teaches you how to love and adore yourself no matter what you've been through, or what's still ahead.

No matter how badly I've been treated, I know this: deep down, I have a good heart. I have true intentions.

And that's something no one can ever take from me.

Your life is your own story to live.

Never give up on building the life you want even if no one else understands it.

Be who *you* want to be, not who others expect you to be.

There's no peace in living for someone else.

Let your mind focus. Let yourself receive positivity.

My hardest moment in life was learning to forgive myself for all the times I doubted my own worth, for every moment I felt afraid, empty, and lost.

Every situation in life is temporary.

When things aren't good, remember it won't last forever.

Better days are coming.

My side of the story may never matter to everyone. That's okay.

Life will go on and I am healing.

I used to be sad about how people treated me.

But then I started to think about how *I* treated them.

Remember the way you treat others is always a reflection of who *you* are.

How others treat you is a reflection of *them,* not your value.

Always remember this:

You're taking your life back.

Love yourself. Respect yourself. Value yourself.

You will forever be your own best friend your number one fan.

As you walk through your story, choose positivity. Believe in yourself.

Someone's actions will always reveal their truth more than their words ever could.

If someone says they care, don't just listen *watch what they do.*

True intentions are shown through consistent effort, not empty promises.

We all go through different kinds of trauma.

If you're a survivor of emotional abuse, know this you already understand what it means to fight battles no one else can see.

The mental, emotional, and physical damage leaves deep marks. You may never fully get over it, but you can stand strong knowing you are worth far more than what broke you.

It took me a while to understand, but I've learned this truth:

If you don't face your demons, they'll end up raising your children.

And you'll be okay with people not knowing your side of the story.

Let them believe what they want. You know your truth.

Believe in yourself now. Stand tall.

Drama will always start small and grow big but act *now.*

Every journey begins with one simple step.

Your dreams might seem out of reach, but every small effort moves you closer to your moment the one that's waiting for *you.*

Every action you take from here brings you closer to your future.

So start today.

Your future self will thank you.